The Microbiome

Richard Lucius

The Microbiome

How our Inner Ecosystem Controls the Immune System and Prevents Inflammation

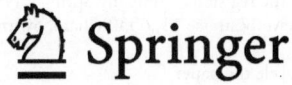

Richard Lucius
Institut für Biologie
Humboldt-Universität zu Berlin
Berlin, Germany

ISBN 978-3-031-78820-8   ISBN 978-3-031-78821-5   (eBook)
https://doi.org/10.1007/978-3-031-78821-5

The original submitted manuscript has been translated into English. The translation was done using artificial intelligence. A subsequent revision was performed by a third party to further refine the work and to ensure that the translation is appropriate concerning content and scientific correctness. It may, however, read stylistically different from a conventional translation.

Translation from the German language edition: "Die Kraft unseres inneren Ökosystems" by Richard Lucius, © Scorpio Verlag in Europa Verlage GmbH, München 2022. Published by Scorpio Verlag. All Rights Reserved.

This Springer imprint is published by the registered company Springer Nature Switzerland AG
The registered company address is: Gewerbestrasse 11, 6330 Cham, Switzerland

If disposing of this product, please recycle the paper.

To Gudrun

Preface

Our immune system, which has evolved over millions of years, is calibrated for a sparse, nature-oriented life. In our modern society, it often goes haywire under the influence of highly processed foods, medications, and lack of contact with a natural environment. The result: More than 25 million people in Germany alone suffer from allergies, autoimmune diseases, and food intolerances that were hardly known in the past. The common denominator of these diseases is chronic inflammatory processes.

It is becoming increasingly clear that our susceptibility to chronic inflammation is largely determined by the bacteria we carry in and on our bodies and with which we come into contact in our environment. We harbor about one kilogram of these inhabitants in our intestines alone. With every breath and every touch of a surface, with every handshake and every kiss, we are exposed to myriads of these tiny creatures.

This microbial world is collectively referred to as the "microbiome." These organisms form an ecosystem within us, in which hundreds of bacterial species cooperate and compete with each other. They metabolize products that humans cannot digest and, in return, provide energy and vital substances. And, much more important than previously thought: They program and control the immune system. Their essential contribution: They inhibit inflammation, so efficiently that they can even mitigate the course of disease in coronavirus infections, which are characterized by inflammatory processes. Only together with our inhabitants do we form a resilient "superorganism."

If we do not take good care of our inner ecosystem, it becomes impoverished and suffers, much like our outer environment, from loss of species. Then, it can no longer protect us from inflammatory diseases. Modern research allows us to analyze the diversity of bacteria and the mechanisms by which they affect us. The result: The human body is in constant exchange with its bacterial environment. We benefit from as large an inner biodiversity as possible. Our sensors register molecules released by bacteria as calming or alarming signals. The way in which our immune system is set depends on the spectrum of microbes that we harbor. This community of microbes is so closely connected to us that they even have a great influence on the formation of our organs, our metabolism, and our cognitive processes. Health is not a primal state, but must be acquired: through harmonious coexistence with the microbiome.

Hunters and gatherers in the Brazilian rainforest, small farmers in Malawi, and traveling horse traders and tinsmiths in Ireland have one thing in common: they all live relatively close to nature. Such people only rarely experience inflammatory diseases. They are constantly in contact with a wide variety of bacteria. Therefore, they harbor a different spectrum of bacterial species and the species diversity of their inner ecosystem is significantly greater than that of, for example, contemporary urban dwellers. Those who, on the other hand, lead a modern life have a depleted microbiome and are more likely to suffer from allergies, autoimmune responses, or food intolerances.

Which factors of the "western lifestyle" are the cause of this phenomenon is still unclear. Is it the highly processed foods, with their excess of sugar, unhealthy fats, salt, emulsifiers, sweeteners, preservatives, or pesticide residues? Is it the excess of antibiotics and other medications? Or the lack of exercise and lack of contact with bacteria from the environment? All these factors, especially diet, have a great influence on the microbiome. They promote the growth of certain types of bacteria and inhibit others, and with each change in the bacterial flora, the natural balance of the immune system also shifts.

With the new research findings on this topic, the possibilities for intervention and the restoration of the lost diversity of our bacterial flora are also growing. For this, we need to have a sensitive balance with our microbiome in mind, always taking our residents into consideration. What do they need to form a diverse ecosystem that harmonizes with our immune system? And what harms them? These questions are particularly important in early childhood, when the microbiome sets the course for later life through epigenetic changes. It is also exciting to learn how a disturbed microbiome and inflammatory diseases are related. Therefore, I include some examples in this book as to how the microbiome, in interaction with the genetic makeup, contributes to the derailment of immune responses and chronic inflammations. The knowledge of how the sensitive balance in our interior works allows for a new understanding of health. This could succeed in dramatically reducing the burden of inflammatory diseases. We should all know that our inner microcosm is a treasure that is endangered by the modern lifestyle and one that we need to handle very carefully.

Berlin, Germany   Richard Lucius

Acknowledgments

I would like to express my sincere thanks to my editor Silke Foos for her dedicated review of the book and helpful comments.

This book would not have been possible without the help of many friends and colleagues, to whom I am deeply grateful. They discussed the concept with me, gave me hints, recommended literature, proofread texts, or were available for interviews. It was fun working with you!

- Prof. Dr. Harri Alenius (Karolinska Institute Stockholm and University of Helsinki)
- Prof. Dr. Karl-Christian Bergmann (Charité University Medicine Berlin)
- Prof. Dr. Michael Blaut (DIfE Potsdam)
- Jörg Blech (DER SPIEGEL)
- Dr. Reinhard Blomert
- Prof. John F. Cryan (University College Cork, Ireland)
- Dr. Tewo Debebe (Biomes World, Wildau)
- Prof. Dr. Andreas Diefenbach (Charité University Medicine Berlin)
- Dr. Rebekka Göpfert
- Prof. Dr. Achim Gruber (Free University of Berlin)
- Prof. Dr. Alf Hamann (German Rheumatism Research Center)
- Dr. Paul Hammer (Biomes World, Wildau)
- Dr. Turid Hammer (The Faroese Hospital, Thorshavn)
- Prof. Dr. Hans Hauner (Technical University of Munich)
- Prof. Dr. Emanuel Heitlinger (Humboldt University of Berlin)
- Prof. Dr. Matthias Hornef (RWTH Aachen)
- Prof. Dr. Urs Jenal (University of Basel)
- Prof. Dr. Malin Johansson (University of Gothenburg)
- Dr. Stefan Jordan (Charité University Medicine Berlin)
- Dr. Gudrun Kochendörfer
- Prof. Dr. Johannes Krause (MPI for Evolutionary Anthropology Leipzig)

- Marlies Kuschel
- Prof. Dr. Matthias Laudes (University Hospital Schleswig-Holstein)
- Prof. Dr. Christian Liedke (Technical University of Munich)
- Prof. Dr. Friedrich Longin (University of Hohenheim)
- Prof. Dr. Charles Mackay (Monash University, Melbourne)
- Dr. Dieter Merkel
- Klaus Michaelis
- Dr. Andrew Moeller (Cornell University, Ithaca, USA)
- Prof. Dr. Erika von Mutius (Helmholtz Center Munich)
- Otto Netzel (Humboldt University of Berlin)
- Prof. Dr. Michael Ohl, Museum of Natural History Berlin)
- Prof. Dr. Friedemann Paul (Charité University Medicine Berlin)
- Prof. Dr. Andreas Pfeiffer (Charité University Medicine Berlin)
- Dr. Norbert Prauser
- Prof. Dr. Alexander Scheffold (University Hospital Schleswig-Holstein)
- Dr. Rainer Schmack
- Laura Schneider
- Prof. Dr. Britta Siegmund (Charité University Medicine Berlin)
- Prof. Dr. Aki Sinkkonen (University of Helsinki)
- Prof. Dr. Uli Steinhoff (University of Marburg)
- Prof. Dr. Alexander Swidsinski (Charité University Medicine Berlin)
- Dr. Wilfried Vahjen (Free University of Berlin)
- Dr. Anna Sofia Veyhe (The Faroese Hospital, Thorshavn)
- Dr. Suvi Virtanen (NIHW Helsinki)
- Prof. Dr. Pal Weihe (The Faroese Hospital, Thorshavn)
- Prof. Dr. Jürgen Zentek (Free University of Berlin)

Contents

1

Allergy & Co.: The New Civilization Diseases

Contents

Inflammatory Diseases, a Modern Epidemic

Spring 2020: Suddenly, the coronavirus pandemic was the number one topic of conversation. With lockdowns, panic-buying and short-time work, it brutally broke into everyday life. Under normal circumstances, diseases are a topic confined to the waiting room of doctor's offices; now, there was hardly a conversation that didn't touch on Corona. The prospect of contracting the life-threatening virus forced everyone to inform and protect themselves. You couldn't simply ignore COVID-19. For the media, the pandemic was a hit: a fresh topic, a plague that could hit anyone. The global significance, coupled with the constant media bombardment, made COVID-19 a societal event, brought new stars and villains to the fore, and led to demonstrations and police operations.

Of course, you talked with friends and acquaintances about how transmission works, how to protect yourself and what to expect in case of an infection. If you wanted to join the conversation, you had to be informed.

Plagues like COVID-19, which fall upon us all of a sudden, get much more attention than chronic diseases, the occurrence of which we have become accustomed to over time. They too can affect millions of people and cause immense suffering but are nevertheless rarely a topic of conversation. They have appeared in less dramatic ways, have rather crept in, and have now become so much a part of daily life that we almost take them for granted. These ailments include diseases that are based on an overreaction of the immune system. Where, in healthy people, the immune system is limited to the defense of pathogens, it also reacts to harmless substances in those affected. Wherever a modern lifestyle spreads around the globe, the frequency of allergies, autoimmune diseases and intolerances to certain foods inevitably increases. And this increase is not due to the rise in the world population or the fact that people are living longer, but rather the more frequent new acquisition of diseases. In Germany, more than a quarter of the population is affected by these "inflammatory diseases". They have dramatically increased in recent decades and, unlike the classic plagues, are an "epidemic of modernity", as a newspaper headline recently declared.

Of these ailments, allergies are the most well-known and widespread. They are, so to speak, the flag bearers of inflammatory diseases, which is why they could be referred to as "Allergy & Co.".

Who had an allergy in the 1960s? I can't remember that there was anyone at my summer camp who couldn't tolerate milk, eggs, or peanuts.

Today, on the other hand, lists circulate in kindergartens of foods that Emma, Ben, Luca, or Mia absolutely must not eat, under threat of an anaphylactic shock. Taking Germany as an example: Currently, almost 19% of all adult citizens suffer from at least one allergy. Additionally, asthma and atopic dermatitis, which are among the allergic diseases in a broader sense, are common and more than 8% of adults and 13% of children, respectively (Bergmann et al. 2016). Much more common than before are severe autoimmune diseases like Type 1 diabetes (0.4%; RKI 2019), chronic intestinal inflammation (0.74%; Hein et al. 2014) and multiple sclerosis (0.3%; Holstiege et al. 2017). It is estimated that up to 30% of the people living in Germany also suffer from digestive disorders, some of which are associated with inflammation, such as celiac disease. These are just a few examples of inflammatory diseases. A complete listing of over 100 ailments would go beyond our scope here.

Science has long sought explanations for this phenomenon, but now it is certain: Our immune system is dependent on contact with our living environment for its functioning. Humans need the right, individually different mixture of microbes on the skin, in the lungs and especially in the gut to stay healthy. Homo sapiens does not live alone, but is rather a "superorganism", which forms a functional unit only together with its inhabitants. Its microbes form a species-rich ecosystem that calms the immune system and protects against overreactions. However, our modern lifestyle has changed both the microbial landscape in our interior and the actual landscape in which we live to such a great degree that it no longer fits our immune system. It is out of balance, raising the alarm for trivial reasons and reacting too strongly. What's behind this?

Our immune cells constantly check every corner of the body, whether there is danger or not. Pathogens such as bacteria, viruses, parasites and fungi contain molecular danger signals that activate the immune system and attract immune cells to the site. Depending on how strong these danger signals are, a decision is made as to whether an attack should take place or not. If it is determined that it should, more immune cells are attracted to the scene and activated, subsequently releasing a cloud of highly reactive chemicals. These substances attack and destroy pathogens, but also damage our own tissue in the process. This attack, which can escalate into a major offensive, is called "inflammation". Inflammations are therefore quite normal, vital reactions. However, the collateral damage is often considerable, so efficient mechanisms of limitation are important.

Harmless substances such as food components or those the body creates on its own normally do not provoke inflammatory responses. They do not stimulate the immune system or even lead to an inhibition of inflammatory reactions through complex mechanisms. A well-balanced immune system thus ignores harmless stimuli or applies the brakes and prevents inflammations.

It is exactly this ability that many people in modern societies have lost. Their immune system also triggers inflammatory reactions against harmless foreign substances such as plant pollen and cannot pause and simply tolerate such substances. The resulting inflammations damage the body's own tissue. Depending on which organ is affected and which type of immune response predominates, very different diseases can occur. Here, a rough distinction is made between allergies, autoimmune diseases, and food intolerances (Table 1.1).

At present, inflammatory diseases are most widespread in the affluent countries of the Western world, but are now increasingly spreading to emerging and developing countries. The reason for the increase is our modern lifestyle, referred to in the specialist literature as the "western lifestyle". This vague term—discussed in more detail in the following chapter—attempts to

Table 1.1 Effects of some inflammatory diseases and their prevalence in Germany

	Effects	Frequency in Germany
Allergic diseases		
Allergies in the strict sense	Temporary inflammatory reactions of mucous membranes and skin	16.6 million[a]
Asthma	Chronic inflammation of the airways, cough	6.57 million[a]
Neurodermatitis	Chronic inflammation of the skin	4.31 million[a]
Autoimmune diseases		
Chronic intestinal inflammations	Massive damage to the intestinal mucosa	615,000[b]
Type-1 diabetes	Destruction of pancreatic cells by inflammation	330,000[c]
Multiple sclerosis	Destruction of nerve cells through inflammation	240,000[d]
Psoriasis	Inflammation of the skin due to misguided immune responses	2.0 million[e]
Rheumatoid arthritis	Inflammation of joints	940,000[f]
Intolerances		
Celiac disease	Digestive problems due to gluten intolerance	830,000[g]
Irritable bowel syndrome	Digestive problems due to food components (FODMAPS)	2.9 to 14 million[h]

[a]Bergmann et al. (2016)
[b]Hein et al. (2014)
[c]RKI (2019)
[d]Holstiege et al. (2017)
[e]Hense et al. (2016)
[f]Sewerin et al. (2019)
[g]Schuppan and Gisbert-Schuppan (2018)
[h]Various sources

summarize the various factors that are typical of the lifestyle of people in modern, affluent societies. The range includes, among other things, nutrition, housing, hygiene, health care, contact with nature, and exercise. For people who still live without the achievements of modern civilization, such as in remote African villages, in the Brazilian rainforest, or even on isolated farms in the mountains, where the Western lifestyle has not yet arrived, inflammatory diseases are virtually unknown.

Many studies show that, for such people living close to nature, contact with microorganisms is an important factor for their health. Their skin, mucous membranes, and intestines are populated by a healthy mixture of many different types of microbes. These microbes, collectively referred to as the "microbiome", form an entire ecosystem in which hundreds of species compete for food and space or cooperate (for the term "microbiome", see the "Microbiome and Microbiota" section on the book's website).

In the intestines of a single adult, there is about one kilogram of bacteria, viruses, parasites, fungi, and archaea (primitive single-celled organisms), including about 40,000,000,000,000 bacteria (in other words: 40 trillion, a number with 13 zeros!). The bacterial cells are thus about as numerous as the cells of the human body, which means that about half our bodies—in terms of the number of cells—is bacteria.

This mass of bacteria lives, consumes energy, and produces substances; it works like an additional organ of our body.

The bacteria defend their territory against intruders, and thus keep disease-causing agents at bay. At the same time, they break down food residues and provide the body with energy, vitamins, and other substances from them. Another important function that has mostly been overlooked: Their metabolic products regulate the immune system, and thus reduce the tendency towards inflammation. Our useful inhabitants are referred to in scientific jargon as "commensals" (Latin: table companions), but they are more than that: Together with our inner ecosystem, we form a powerful superorganism, as long as the balance between the partners is right.

In contrast to people living close to nature, the biodiversity of this inner ecosystem in modern city dwellers has declined significantly due to unhealthy diet, excessive use of medication, and lack of exercise. Environmental chemicals, pesticides, food additives, and many other factors also have an impact on our microbial landscape. Thus, the balance between the species has been substantially disturbed and bacteria have spread that were previously rare, while others have disappeared. Much like humans ruin their external environment through reckless overuse, they also abuse their inner ecosystem through the modern lifestyle. Such a depleted and altered microbiome cannot fulfill its diverse tasks and is also not able to keep inflammatory responses in check.

The Worldwide Increase in Allergy & Co.

The increase in inflammatory diseases is a global trend that first appeared in industrialized countries but is now increasingly affecting emerging and developing countries. Even in the most remote corners of the earth, such as New Guinea, an increase in these diseases is observed as soon as people connect to the modern world (Herbert et al. 2009). Within a few years, the diet, medical care, living situation, and many other factors change. With this "Western lifestyle", which will be explained in detail later, civilization diseases occur.

The large-scale increase in inflammatory diseases, from Europe to the USA, from Japan to Australia, began between 1960 and 1970 and has accelerated since the 1980s and 1990s. In Europe, the Scandinavian countries are particularly affected, while development in the Eastern European countries was slower during socialism. There, the lifestyle changed less and, accordingly, the increase in inflammatory diseases was also more moderate. In some industrialized countries, the curves are no longer rising, but have reached a plateau. A possible reason: By now, more or less all individuals who are particularly susceptible to inflammatory diseases due to their genetic makeup have fallen ill, so there is no further increase. If essentially only the offspring fall ill, the number of new cases each year remains relatively stable.

The same trend is now being observed in emerging countries like China, India, and South Africa, albeit with a time delay. Asia is catching up particularly quickly, in some cases, with extremely high growth rates.

For example, a 30-fold increase (!!) in inflammatory bowel disease was reported from Hong Kong over a period of 30 years (Ng et al. 2017). In developing countries, the values are still very low in some cases, but they are rising with the transition to modern living conditions. However, it is not only chronic intestinal inflammations that have seen this increase; they are just a particularly good example because they are so noticeable and burdensome that they are quite well systematically recorded and researched. The same trend is also followed by most other inflammatory diseases.

With the spread of the Western lifestyle, the frequency of inflammatory diseases in emerging and developing countries will continue to increase in the coming years and decades. It is foreseeable that, even in regions with previously low rates, the number of diseases will continue to rise until saturation is reached at a similarly high level as that in industrialized countries.

With this pattern of spread, inflammatory diseases are a real pandemic, a worldwide epidemic. The data is alarming! However, it is not easy to filter out the relevant information from the multitude of different studies and put together a coherent picture. A major challenge is to bring the numerous different inflammatory diseases under a common denominator. After all, the corresponding publications usually emphasize the peculiarities of diseases and differentiate them from each other, rather than highlighting the commonalities. For example, type 1 diabetes and multiple sclerosis, which demonstrate very different clinical pictures, have a common root, namely an increased propensity for inflammation.

One especially encounters problems when one wants to track how the frequency of such diseases has developed over decades. At the time of the first description of diseases that were once rare and are now common, hardly anyone suspected how significant they could become. Accordingly, solid base-line data is lacking for many inflammatory diseases. The safest method for generating data that is reliable at all is a continuous, long-term recording of all disease cases with standardized diagnostic methods. Such far-reaching long-term studies and the corresponding registers unfortunately only exist in a few countries with highly developed health systems, such as in Scandinavia.

From the information in such disease registers, the incidence (number of new cases) and prevalence (total number of cases) of diseases in a population can be calculated. If there are no continuously maintained registers, one is dependent on data from individual studies, which, however, are often not precisely comparable with each other, because, for example, the methods used are slightly different. Data from several studies are often summarized in "meta-studies". Such overviews are extremely helpful, because they often capture older and less accessible literature, thus providing a good overall picture.

One such convincing meta-study comes from Loftus (2004), which shows the worldwide increase in the incidence of chronic intestinal inflammations in the second half of the twentieth century based on seven long-term studies (Fig. 1.1). All curves run in the same direction. This graphic shows—like the

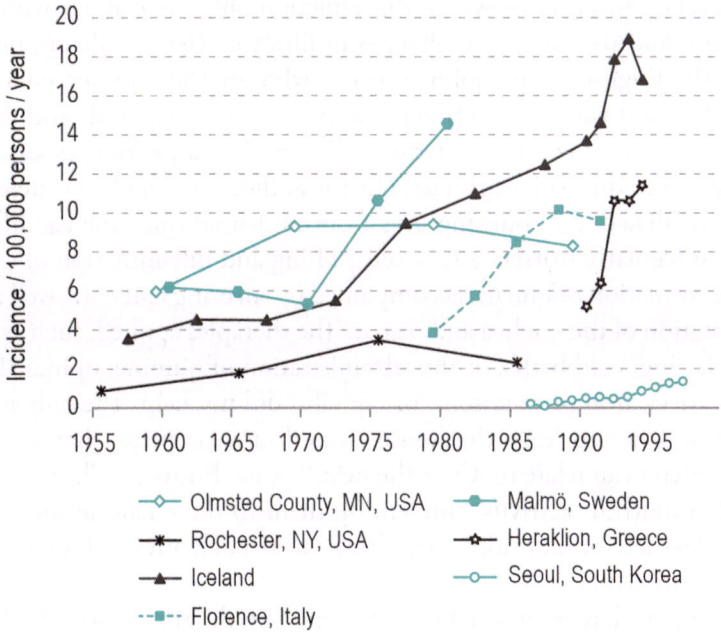

Fig. 1.1 Increase in new cases of ulcerative colitis in various countries with a Western lifestyle (cases/100,000 people/year). (From Loftus 2004. © Scorpio Verlag in Europa Verlage GmbH, München. Reproduced with permission)

results of many other meta-studies—that, without a doubt, new cases have indeed increased significantly during the period shown.

The Example of Allergies

The rise of inflammatory diseases in industrialized countries can best be traced through allergies. These conditions are particularly suitable for demonstrating the link between Western lifestyle and the increase in inflammatory diseases, as the data on them is the most extensive available.

When we think of allergies, hay fever often comes to mind first. In Germany, every seventh adult and every tenth child suffers from this affliction, caused by pollen from grasses and other plants (Bergmann et al. 2016). Those affected react to pollen contact with sneezing, swollen nasal mucous membranes, tearing eyes, conjunctivitis, and coughing, not to mention the associated drowsiness. Also: allergies that have started as hay fever in the nose can, over time, also affect the lower respiratory tract and develop into asthma. This progression is so typical that it is referred to as "allergic march."

We have become so accustomed to hay fever that we now mostly consider it a natural occurrence. However, this affliction only came about with industrialization and the associated changes in lifestyle. The first description goes back to the English doctor John Bostock, who, in 1809, presented a case of "Catarrhus aestivus", or summer catarrh, to the Medical and Surgical Association in London, of the patient JB, who had a periodic disease of the eyes and chest. This patient JB (actually the author himself) had suffered from tearing, reddened, and burning eyes from mid-June since the age of 8. His condition regularly worsened to severe itching and inflammation of the eyes, with the formation of mucus, accompanied by sneezing and narrowed airways with irritation of the trachea and throat. The therapies applied, such as bloodletting, fasting, cold baths, or the administration of quinine, opium (!), mercury, laxatives, iron preparations, or digitalis, did not help. The only relieving measure was not to leave the house. A perfect description that any pollen allergy sufferer can relate to. Over the next 9 years, Bostock collected 28 more cases of "Catarrhus aestivus", presenting them to the scientific society in an essay, and is therefore considered the first describer of hay fever (Ramachandran and Aronson 2011).

In Germany, hay fever was first mentioned by the spa doctor Dr. Alfter in Bad Oeynhausen, who, in 1855, reported on a patient who had regularly suffered from rhinitis, conjunctivitis, and shortness of breath "at the time when the rye blooms" since his seventh year of life. He noted: "The sea air ... was only really effective when the wind came from the sea." In 1862, Philipp Phoebus, in Giessen, collected cases from all over Europe in a first standard work and mentioned, as a special feature, that the frequency was "strikingly low" and that the disease occurred "more often in the wealthy, educated.." (quoted from Bergmann 2019).

It took another decade to find the cause of hay fever: In his book "Experimental Researches on the Causes and Nature of Catarrhus Aestius" (1873), the British doctor Charles Blackley, also a hay fever sufferer, describes a variety of experiments to trigger the allergic reaction in the laboratory. He achieved the most reliable results with pollen. He tested pollen from no fewer than 74 plant species and found that he could trigger the most severe reactions with grass pollen. Sun and heat, on the other hand, had no effect. Furthermore, he also noticed that the disease had been much less common 15–20 years earlier and was virtually unknown before that. He found that hay fever would mainly occur in the educated class of the population, especially among lawyers and theologians. In contrast, hardly any farmer was found to suffer from it, even though they were most exposed to pollen. His conclusion: The state acquired through mental work is probably a prerequisite for the development of hay fever. The increase would be associated with increasing urbanization, which would promote civilization and education. Indeed, England was the pioneer of industrialization and urbanization in Europe, while the other countries of Europe were still predominantly agricultural in the 1850s.

Hay fever as a disease of the educated: This view held for a long time in England. People suffered, but also felt superior to the "lower classes". Sir Morell McKenzie, a famous English physician, stated, in the paper "Hay Fever and Paroxysmal Sneezing" (1889), that the disease was almost exclusively limited to cultivated individuals and that the tendency to hay fever was linked to one's intellectual level. This fit well with the fact that men are significantly more affected than women, which he pointed out to advocates of equality. He considered the fact that hay fever was almost exclusively known in England and the USA as a sign of the superiority of the "English race". He even fantasized that sneezing could become a test "to distinguish the chosen from the common herd".

Affluent pollen allergy sufferers could at least temporarily escape their disease by spending the pollen season at seaside or mountain resorts. Thus, in some regions, a veritable tourism developed where one met one's peers in an upscale environment during "hayfever holidays". Among wealthy Britons, Heligoland, which was a British crown colony until 1890, was a popular refuge. The isolated island far out in the North Sea still promotes its pollen-poor air and places ads as an "allergy-friendly community".

A survey from Switzerland in 1926 showed a hay fever prevalence of only about 1% at that time. In the tone of his English colleagues, the author of this study (Rehsteiner 1926) also speaks of a disease of the educated, in which "twenty times more hay fever patients fall on the 'head workers' than on the total population". A study from 1958 shows a prevalence of about 5% in Switzerland. This trend continued with an increase to 9.5% (1985) and then about 14% (1991). A compilation published in 2017 mentions a hay fever prevalence of about 20% in Switzerland (Ballmer-Weber and Heibling 2017).

The rate of hay fever in Switzerland has thus increased 20fold in just under 100 years! From a rare disease, it has become an affliction that now affects about one in five citizens. The situation is similar in Germany, where the Robert Koch Institute spoke, in 2017, of a "tsunami that will overwhelm us" (Fig. 1.2).

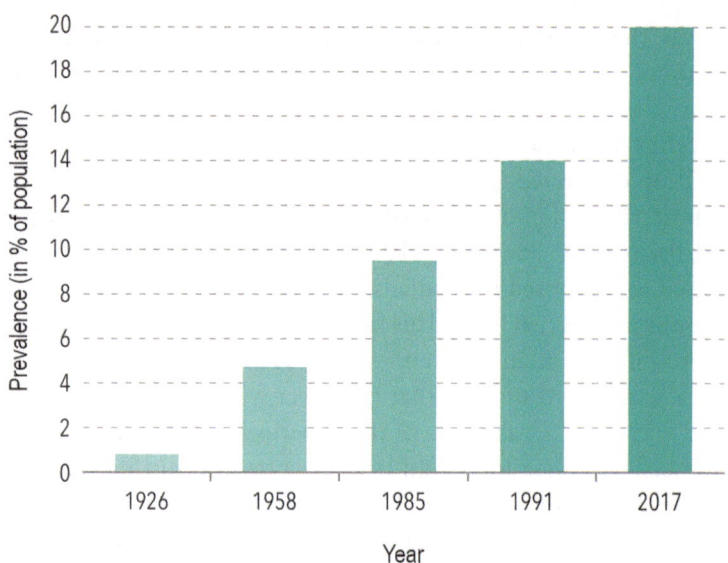

Fig. 1.2 Increase in the prevalence of hay fever in Switzerland, in % of the population. Combined from various sources. (Rehsteiner 1926; Schnyder 1958; Wüthrich et al. 1986; SAPALDIA 1991; Ballmer-Weber and Heibling 2017. © Scorpio Verlag in Europa Verlage GmbH, München. Reproduced with permission)

Inflammation and Immune Tolerance

The problem with allergy sufferers is that contact with otherwise harmless substances triggers inflammation. The term "inflammation" essentially means that the immune system flexes its muscles: immune cells are activated by a stimulus and attract other immune cells with messenger substances, which then take action and attack. Inflammations are vital to the repelling of pathogens, but they also always damage the body itself. The spectrum of inflammation ranges from potentially deadly appendicitis and pneumonia to the subliminal reactions that even doctors can only identify through markers in the blood.

Just as important as inflammatory processes are mechanisms that ensure that the processes that have started are switched off again, that an anti-inflammation, so to speak, takes place. In this process, reaction cascades are actively downregulated by messenger substances and contacts between cells. One could speak of a brake that ensures that harmless stimuli do not lead to a chain reaction and the associated destruction.

Immunology summarizes these processes with the term "immune tolerance". This word is a key term for understanding inflammatory diseases and one of the main content focuses of this book. Influences of the Western lifestyle have weakened immune tolerance in many people. This leads to different diseases, but they all have a similar trigger underlying them, namely, an increased propensity for inflammation. These inflammatory diseases develop less dramatically than, for example, COVID-19 and they do not kill directly, but they significantly impair the affected individuals and pave the way for many other ailments.

Everyone knows such acute inflammations as are caused by a foreign body, like a splinter that has torn into one's flesh. The surrounding skin becomes red, swells and hurts. What happens in detail? Cells of the immune system, which patrol within the tissue, are alerted and activated by injury signals and by molecules of bacteria that adhere to the splinter. These molecular danger signals have a key function: the cells immediately release messenger substances that attract other immune cells from the surrounding tissue and from blood vessels. These crawl over to the site of the injury, pour out a whole cocktail of aggressive chemicals, and produce, among other things, free radicals that kill the bacteria. More cells are attracted, and the process escalates. This results in a major attack, in which many body cells also die. The attack only comes to a halt and repair mechanisms kick in when the splinter is removed, and the last bacteria are destroyed.

A similar activation of the immune system also initially starts when immune cells react to weaker stimuli. A multitude of such weakly activating events occurs every day, as a result of contact with foreign substances such as pollen or food components, but also because of changes in one's own bodily substances or simply immune cells triggering a false alarm. If, however, during this initial activation of the immune system, strong danger signals are missing, such as components of pathogens, braking responses of immune tolerance come into play and stop the reaction before major damage occurs.

An optimally adjusted immune system thus accelerates with strong stimuli such as pathogens, but brakes with weak stimuli such as pollen or food components, bringing the reaction to a halt. In healthy people, therefore, only relevant triggers cause the immune system to riot. If the immune brake fails due to disturbed immune tolerance, however, inflammations smolder and can easily flare up with further stimuli and develop into an acute inflammation. Where these "silent inflammations" take place determines which diseases occur. For example, in allergies and intestinal inflammations, the mucous membranes are affected, in rheumatoid arthritis, the joints, in type 1 diabetes, the pancreas, and in multiple sclerosis, the nervous system.

The advertised message of many pharmaceutical companies that a strong immune system is the best way to health is therefore incorrect in its simplicity. As the example of allergies shows, strong immune responses are not always positive; many patients would be glad if they had weaker inflammatory responses, at least during the pollen season. It's not about a strong immune system, but rather a very well-balanced one. A functioning immune tolerance is extremely important!

The Quantum Leap of Biomedicine

Events such as the discovery of penicillin or the deciphering of the human genome are so significant that they have not only shaped medicine, but also influenced and continue to influence society as a whole. Mostly unnoticed, we are currently experiencing upheavals in biomedicine that will have equally far-reaching consequences.

On the one hand, new DNA sequencing techniques became available in the 2000s and quickly conquered the market. Compared to old methods, genes can now be analyzed at 200 million times the speed using high-throughput sequencing. While the sequencing of the first human genome took 10 years and kept 10,000 researchers busy, machines now take less than a day to accomplish the same thing. With its new techniques, science has vehemently tackled the microbiome, an issue that could not be tackled before due to its extreme complexity. What was found was breathtaking: The skin, the mucous membranes, and, especially, the human gut are densely populated by hundreds of microbial species. We are now beginning to understand how individual species of bacteria influence immune responses, metabolism, and even moods, with certain molecules.

On the other hand, immunology has developed into a molecular science over the past few decades. Where, in the past, one was limited to looking at and counting immune cells under a microscope, today, the interactions of those cells can be precisely described at the molecular level and modern drugs allow for targeted interventions in these processes. While treatments were once limited to symptoms, thanks to the findings of modern immunology, inflammation is now tackled directly at the root. If you specifically block certain communication pathways between immune cells, inflammation signals are switched off and the situation calms down. Immunology and microbiome research are thus, for the first time, getting to the root causes of inflammatory diseases. A paradigm shift is taking place: once, one could only observe and describe; today, one can fathom molecular details and intervene in processes.

The new techniques of biomedicine show that humans and their microbes are closely intertwined, that both partners only function well together. The microbiome influences the tendency to inflammation and many other characteristics of ours to an extent never before suspected. Bacteria and other microorganisms balance our immune system so that inflammatory responses to food components and other harmless substances are downregulated, while, at the same time, dangerous pathogens can be attacked. This interaction works because humans and their microbes have undergone millions of years of co-evolution, from which both sides benefit.

Exciting Perspectives

Inflammatory diseases are a massive problem, but, as a whole, society has barely grasped it. The industry, on the other hand, has understood its economic significance for a long time. "If I add up all autoimmune disorders, (...) the field of these diseases represents the largest pharmaceutical market in the world. The best-selling drug worldwide, the monoclonal antibody Humira, which targets the inflammation-promoting cytokine TNF-α and is used against half a dozen autoimmune diseases, generates more than 15 billion dollars in sales annually," says Stephane Boissel, CEO of the France-based company TxCell. This is the industry's perspective. The antibody actually achieved sales of 20.69 billion US dollars in 2021 (Statista 2021). However, the market for the entire group of biologicals, the modern remedies against inflammatory diseases, is much larger. Combined, their annual sales amount to about 221 billion US dollars (Statista 2020). The medications for a single patient cost up to 20,000 Euros per year.

Since chronic inflammatory diseases usually need to be treated for life, the medications are a steadily flowing source of profits for the pharmaceutical companies that develop and market them. From the perspective of the patient and the taxpayer, it would be much more desirable to permanently restore the immune balance disturbed by our modern life. Successful prophylaxis brings health at a fraction of the costs caused by the disease. If it were possible to reduce the frequency of inflammatory diseases, many people would be better off and the stressed healthcare systems would simultaneously be massively relieved.

Why is there still hardly any public awareness of inflammatory diseases? It cannot be due to a lack of economic significance. One difficulty probably lies in seeing the various inflammatory diseases as a unit, because, despite their common root, they are very different. Who realizes that ailments such as allergies and multiple sclerosis have inflammation as a common denominator? Who is aware that the more than 100 different inflammatory diseases, despite all their differences, have common features? Even in medicine, this awareness is not very pronounced, because these ailments have only been considered together since around the 2000s. In the statistics, the individual diseases are each listed separately, but not summarized. Thus, even allergies, the largest group of inflammatory diseases, do not make it into the list of the ten most important reasons for a doctor's visit in Germany (which is led by back pain). However, if one were to understand the inflammatory diseases as a unit, because their common cause is an exaggerated tendency towards inflammation, their significance would be much clearer.

Even though we only understand individual facets of the interaction between microbiome and immune response so far, understanding is growing rapidly, not least because of the technical advances in molecular biology, biomedicine, and data processing. The range of these new insights is enormous, and it is clear that a new door is opening in medicine, with new opportunities for prevention and healing. The trend towards personalized medicine opens up completely new perspectives here as well. Many researchers have the goal of equipping patients with a customized microbiome based on individual genome data. Personalized cocktails of commensal bacteria, along with other health services, could create a new, lucrative field of activity for the booming health and wellness industry. But we should not wait for this, rather taking the initiative to improve the disturbed cooperation with our commensals through healthy lifestyle and nutrition ourselves!

References

Ballmer-Weber B, Helbling A (2017) Allergische Rhinitis. Swiss Med Forum 17:179–186

Bergmann KC (2019) Sind wir bald alle betroffen? Neue Daten zur Entwicklung von Allergien in Deutschland? Lecture in Hanover

Bergmann KC et al (2016) aktueller Stand zur Verbreitung von Allergien in Deutschland. Allergo J Int 25:6–10

Hein R et al (2014) Prevalence of inflammatory bowel disease: estimates for 2010 and trends in Germany from a large insurance-based regional cohort. Scand J Gastroenterol 49:1325–1335

Hense S et al (2016) Prävalenz der Rheumatoiden Arthritis in Deutschland auf Basis von Kassendaten. Regionale Unterschiede und erste Ergebnisse der PROCLAIR-Studie. Z Rheumatol 75:819–827

Herbert O et al (2009) Western lifestyle and increased prevalence of atopic diseases. An example from a small Papuan and New Guinean Island. WAO J 2:130–137

Holstiege J et al (2017) Epidemiologie der MS. Eine populationsbasierte deutschlandweite Studie. Zentralinstitut für kassenärztliche Versorgung in Deutschland. Versorgungsbericht No. 17/09. Berlin. https://doi.org/10.20364/VA-17.09

Loftus EV (2004) Clinical epidemiology of inflammatory bowel disease: incidence, prevalence, and environmental influences. Gastroenterology 126:1504–1517

Ng SC et al (2017) Worldwide incidence and prevalence of inflammatory bowel disease in the 21st century: a systematic review of population-based studies. Lancet 390:2769–2778

Ramachandran M, Aronson JK (2011) John Bostock's first description of hayfever. J R Soc Med 104:237–240

Rehsteiner R (1926) Schweiz Z Gesdheitspfl 6:3, cited in Doerr, R. (1944) In: Konstitution-Idiosynkrasien, Stoffwechel und Ernährung. Springer-Verlag OHG, Berlin

RKI (2019) Diabetestypen sind nicht auf Altersgruppen beschränkt: Typ-1-Diabetes bei Erwachsenen und Typ-2-Diabetes bei Kindern und Jugendlichen. J Health Monitor 4(2)

Schnyder UW (1958) Zur Allergologie und Familienpathologie der Allergien. Dermatologica 116:283–289

Schuppan D, Gisbert-Schuppan K (2018) Tägliches Brot: Krank durch Weizen, Gluten und ATI. Springer-Verlag GmbH

Sewerin P et al (2019) Prevalence and incidence of psoriasis and psoriatic arthritis. Ann Rheum Dis 78:286–287

Statista   (2020).   https://de.statista.com/statistik/daten/studie/297580/umfrage/weltweiter-umsatz-mit-biologicals. Accessed 12 Nov 2022

Statista   (2021).   https://de.statista.com/statistik/daten/studie/547194/umfrage/umsatz-des-pharmaunternehmens-abbvie-mit-dem-arzneimittel-humira. Accessed 27 Feb 2022

Wüthrich B et al (1986) Incidence of pollinosis in Switzerland. Results of a representative demographic survey with consideration of other allergic disorders. Schweiz Med Wochenschr 116:109–117

2

How Our Life Has Changed

Contents

The Iron Curtain: Ticket for Time Travel

Science has long barely noticed the alarming increase in inflammatory diseases. This is not too surprising, because differences are best recognized when comparisons can be made. Contrasts catch the eye, but a continuous increase from a low level, as with the inflammatory diseases, easily escapes attention. Inflammatory diseases were so rare for such a long time that they were not on the screen. They are also not directly fatal and not contagious, which is why they also remained under the radar of doctors.

The increase in inflammatory diseases between 1960 and 1980 in many countries was so strong then that it could hardly be overlooked. When the Iron Curtain fell in 1989 and the division of Europe ended, it was noticed that inflammatory diseases in the former Soviet sphere of influence were nowhere near as common as in the capitalist West. In the East, economic development had progressed much more slowly than in the West and the standard of living was accordingly lower. There, time had, so to speak, stood still. The Iron Curtain had created the possibility of time travel between the 1990s (in the West) and the 1960s (in the East)! Comparisons of the ways of life in the West and East could provide clues to the causes of the increase. So, people began to compare living conditions in the West and East and to check their relevance for inflammatory diseases.

Particularly good conditions for such comparisons were found in Northern Europe: Finland, long a pawn of political interests, was formerly occupied by both Russia and Sweden at different times. Part of the former Finnish peninsula of Karelia, not far from St. Petersburg, remained with the Soviet Union in the course of the poker game of the occupying powers over the distribution of territories and is now part of Russia. The population on both sides of the border has the same roots, so genetically determined differences in the occurrence of diseases do not play a role. The climate and environmental conditions are also comparable in both parts of Karelia.

However, the living conditions in both areas could hardly be more different: While Finland has a highly developed infrastructure and one of the highest per capita incomes in Europe, the population in the Russian part of Karelia lived under similarly poor conditions as those in the post-war period when the Iron Curtain fell. On the Scandinavian side, urbanization had made rapid progress, while in the Russian part of the region, people maintained their small-scale farming lifestyle. While the Scandinavians had access to all the achievements of modern life and consumer society from the 1960s onwards, scarcity was the norm on the side of the border living under socialism. Hardly any number can express this better than the gross national product: In 2001, the annual economic output on the Finnish side was 25,130 US dollars per person, while it was 1660 US dollars on the Russian side, less than a tenth. Even today, life there is more modest: Food is partly supplied from home gardens, people cook for themselves, live with several generations in modest houses and keep more pets. In this border region, therefore, the computer age and subsistence economy meet in a confined space.

These conditions in Karelia, a genetically similar population on both sides of the border, but with very different living conditions, were ideal for detailed investigations into the cause of inflammatory diseases. Even on the drawing board, one could hardly have found a better design for a study. Therefore, in 1989, after the fall of the Iron Curtain, in cooperation with Finnish and Russian doctors, cohorts of children were formed who were followed for years in terms of their lifestyle and the occurrence of type 1 diabetes, celiac disease, inflammatory bowel disease, and allergies. The differences found could hardly be more drastic: Finland had the highest per capita prevalence of type 1 diabetes in Europe, while the corresponding frequency in the Russian part of Karelia was only about 15% of this value. The rate of celiac disease, caused by intolerance to the gluten protein of cereals, also differed: Here, the disease rates in the Finnish part of the region were about five times higher than in the Russian part. Allergy tests also showed similar results, with three to five times more children in the Finnish area showing IgE antibodies, a marker for allergic sensitization (Kondrashova et al. 2012). Hay fever and peanut allergy, the most common allergic diseases in Finland, were virtually non-existent in the Russian part of Karelia (Rukolainen et al. 2017).

What was the reason for these differences? Did certain conditions in Russia protect against inflammatory diseases or did risk factors in Finland cause these ailments? As a source of potential hazards from the Western lifestyle, diet, hygiene, drug use, and many other factors were considered, but the focus was initially on infections. Indeed, the medical histories of the children showed a propensity for infections: For example, 73% of the Russian children had an infection with Helicobacter pylori, a bacterium that usually does not cause diseases and downregulates inflammatory responses but can cause stomach ulcers and stomach cancer. In contrast, only 5% of Finnish children were infected with the pathogen. Similar was the case with infections by the Hepatitis A virus, diarrhea-causing viruses and with the parasite Toxoplasma gondii. Infections with parasitic worms were also much more common in the Russian part than in Finland.

This suggested that either the infections themselves had a protective effect or the living conditions under which one acquires infections were responsible for the protection. Further studies pointed to the importance of such accompanying circumstances: Dust from households in the Russian part had a different composition of bacterial species, including a seven-times-higher proportion of bacteria that also live in or on animals (Kondrashova et al. 2012). In addition, microbiome studies showed differences in the composition of the gut flora of toddlers in the Finnish and Russian parts of Karelia. It was suspected that the gut flora of the Russian children had a calming effect on their immune systems, so they developed immune responses to harmless substances less often than the little Finns (Vatanen et al. 2016). This Karelia study will be further discussed in more detail later in the context of type 1 diabetes, because, here, for the first time, mechanisms were demonstrated that lead to immune tolerance in early childhood, and thus shape the risk of disease in later life.

The connection between lifestyle and the frequency of inflammatory diseases in the Finnish-Russian border region was an eye-opener for critics who doubted the increase in diseases in modern societies. However, the epidemiological studies in Karelia only described correlations of disease frequency and lifestyle, but could not establish causal relationships. After all, a high density of storks in an area with high numbers of children does not prove that the stork brings the children. But: The epidemiological data provided the impetus to experimentally investigate the causes of disease frequency in animal models and to further deepen the relationships in molecular studies. Thus, the Karelia studies are crucial for understanding inflammatory diseases. They showed that a major factor in their development is the Western lifestyle.

Similar, albeit less pronounced differences in the frequency of inflammatory diseases were also evident in the East and West regions of the formerly divided Germany after the fall of the Berlin Wall. Here, too, during the division into two states from 1945 to 1989, the social systems had developed differently, leading to differences in lifestyle and consumption habits. The differences were most pronounced in allergic diseases, i.e., pollen allergy (= hay fever), asthma, and atopic dermatitis.

For people born before 1960 (who were 30 years or older at the time of the fall of the Berlin Wall), the frequency of allergic diseases did not differ significantly between East and West Germans. These people had spent their childhood and youth under similarly modest (and microbe-rich) post-war conditions and their immune systems had been similarly programmed. For those born after 1960, the trend was clear: Those who grew up in the socialist East system had significantly less pollen allergy or asthma than someone who spent their childhood and youth in the capitalist West (Krämer et al. 2014).

Apparently, the consumer society of the West that emerged since the 1960s led to a higher risk of allergic diseases. Those born and raised there had a higher disease risk compared to the average East German. After reunification, the frequency of allergic diseases in both parts of Germany slowly increased. Among children born in East Germany after the fall of the Berlin Wall, who increasingly grew up in a consumer society, the frequency quickly increased. About 10 years after the fall of the Wall, the "western lifestyle" had become so prevalent in the former East that the risk for those born then was the same in both parts of Germany (von Mutius et al. 1998).

Between Abundance and Stress:
The "Western lifestyle"

What is this "Western lifestyle" that is causing the number of inflammatory diseases to rise? There is no universally valid definition of the term and it is difficult to define, as one needs a word that characterizes the typical way of life of people in modern, mostly urban societies. But even in highly developed industrial countries, people live very differently. Just think of people in Great Britain compared to those in Japan, with their different eating habits and leisure activities. In addition, the individual differences within a society are enormous:

Couch potatoes and sports fans, vegetarians and carnivores, nature freaks and city dwellers, all these very different characters embody a western lifestyle. But where is the common denominator that applies to the majority of the population in industrial countries? What matters? Inevitably, the term "Western lifestyle" remains rather vague.

The characteristics of our modern life are achievements that are taken for granted in today's Central Europe: We use germ-free drinking water and flush toilets, refrigerators, microwaves and freezers, washing machines and vacuum cleaners. Hygiene is a priority. Changes in the world of work have led to a decrease in outdoor physical labor, replaced by sedentary activities—often in front of a screen. Despite these achievements, which actually make life easier, the stress level has increased, because we are more tightly scheduled and flooded with information. Modern humans mostly stay indoors, move little and have relatively little contact with soil, plants and animals. We no longer grow vegetables and fruits in our home gardens, with a large percentage of our diet now consisting of (agro)industrially produced foods from the supermarket. We enjoy medical care that, thanks to antibiotics and vaccinations, has led to a decrease in infectious diseases and a significantly extended life expectancy.

The roots of the "western lifestyle", which now prevails in all developed industrial nations, have a lot to do with societal changes that, in particular, swept over from America after the Second World War, when politics and culture in the Western part of Europe increasingly oriented themselves towards the USA. From there, consumption and lifestyle habits were adopted; fast food, blue jeans and television series spread, along with a new sense of life. No wonder, then, that the Anglo-American world was often and still is a pioneer in terms of inflammatory diseases.

But which individual aspects could be responsible for this immune dysregulation? How have the details of our daily life changed since the post-war period, since the 1960s and 1970s? How have the worlds of work and leisure behavior, environment and nature, nutrition, hygiene and all the many other factors that make up lifestyle changed? The best way to trace the possible causes of the epidemic of inflammatory diseases is to briefly review the most striking changes in lifestyle.

The Change in the World of Work and Leisure

In the period after the Second World War, when inflammatory diseases were still rare, the focus in Europe was initially mainly on reconstruction. Especially in Germany, it was necessary to re-enable life in the completely destroyed cities and to get the economy going. About 8 million displaced people were looking for a new home and work. In the Western part of Europe, the economy quickly got back on its feet, especially in Germany and Austria, where the upswing happened so quickly that the term "economic miracle" became a catchphrase. Germany developed into a successful export nation, so that purchasing power increased and the gross national product tripled by 1960.

This development has completely changed the world of work. As late as 1949, about 21% of the population in Germany worked in agriculture, mostly on small farms. This number quickly decreased in favor of industrial jobs and dropped to just 1.4% by 2020. Manual labor predominated until the 1960s, for example, in manufacturing and construction. But soon, labor-saving technologies led to a decline in manual labor. At the same time, in most professions, the everyday occasions for movement, which are essential for a healthy life, decreased. This trend was further exacerbated by the increase in screen work. In 2016, two out of every three employees worked mainly at sedentary workplaces (TK Movement Study 2016). Also, the commute to work is usually done sitting in a car, train, or bus, while, in the past, distances were shorter and people often walked or cycled (ADAC Mobility Study 2010). While, in 1950, about 10 km were covered on foot on an average working day, an average office worker today only takes about 1500 steps a day, corresponding to a distance of 975 m.

It would be healthy to compensate for this lack of movement in working life through an increase in physical activity and sports in leisure time. The truth is far from this: The sitting marathon at work continues in leisure time. In a study by the Techniker health insurance, 42% of respondents said they were a couch potato in the evening and hung around on the sofa. "Sitting, staring, resting"—this is how the study summarized it, drastically, but correctly (TK Mobility Study 2016). Other studies report that middle-aged people typically spend 23 h a day in a resting position. The trend towards little movement also affects young people, as 89% of the age group from 10 to 19 years are online every day and spend an average of 205 min a day consuming media (JIM Study 2019). Shopping, errands and visits are increasingly done by car, instead of walking or cycling. The average citizen is a couch potato, even if health-conscious, young joggers and spry retirees in the parks suggest a different picture.

Everything Germ-Free: Hygiene

Since the end of the nineteenth century, medicine has increasingly shaped the awareness that cleanliness is vital to prevent infectious diseases. The more it became clear that infections are caused by bacteria, viruses, or parasites, the more efficient methods of disinfection and infection prophylaxis were established in the first half of the twentieth century in the medical field, with a corresponding increasingly pronounced awareness of hygiene in people's personal lives as well. Nevertheless, hygiene in the 1960s had not yet penetrated all areas of life as deeply as it has today.

Let's take milk as an example, a product that we now know almost exclusively as a carton-wrapped rectangular drink. At large dairy farms in 2021, the cows enter a milking parlor several times a day, where a robotic arm cleans the udder and attaches the milking equipment to then draw off the milk. The turbo cows, fed with silage and concentrated feed, give about twice as much milk as in 1970. The milk is immediately cooled and then brought by the collection truck to the dairy, without breaking the cold chain. This way, the number of bacteria in the milk, a quality feature, which also determines the producer price, is kept low. "Fresh milk" is then pasteurized (heated to 72–75 °C for 15–20 s) to reduce the number of germs. It can also be heated more intensely for a short time to then be sold as a "longer lasting" product. However, most Germans prefer UHT milk, which is completely germ-free, and thus very long-lasting, due to brief heating to 135–150 °C.

What a difference from the past: Until the 1960s, milking was still done by hand. The milk was collected in cans, taken to the dairy, processed, and from there again distributed in cans to the milk shops. The customer collected the open milk with their own container, the liquid shooting out in full stream from the hand-operated pump in the milk shop. This product was not pasteurized, and therefore contained many bacteria. If you filled a bowl with milk in the summer and left it on the windowsill, it turned into a delicious, sour-tasting curdled milk within a day. The lactic acid bacteria that had gotten into the milk during the production process and multiplied were responsible for this. So, for dinner, you had a hefty dose of probiotic bacteria, without having to buy a dietary supplement at the pharmacy. With today's boxed product, you can no longer make curdled milk, because it does not contain enough suitable bacteria to sour the milk.

Similarly, quality standards have also changed in other areas of food production. Today, fruits and vegetables mostly come from large farms that, from the outset, use optimized methods to keep dirt at bay. In the past, you had to wash lettuce at least twice to avoid getting sand between your teeth, but today, you can more or less blindly chop the lettuce hearts from the cellophane packaging into the bowl. Of course, along with the sand, the bacteria have also decreased, and with the cleanliness, the transmission of parasitic worms has largely come to a halt. The post-war generation is probably the first generation to grow up almost without parasitic worms. Similarly, other former common diseases, such as tuberculosis, and childhood viral infections, such as mumps, measles and chickenpox, have been massively suppressed thanks to hygiene measures, antibiotics, and vaccinations. Flush toilets, vacuum cleaners, steam mops, and disinfectants make life difficult for pathogens, but they also eradicate harmless environmental bacteria. The Corona pandemic has shown us how important it is to prevent infections through appropriate measures. However, we must not lose sight of the fact that our microbiome constantly needs replenishment from the outside. If this exchange is lacking, our inner ecosystem becomes impoverished and the balance of the immune system is endangered. As beneficial as the improvements in hygiene are, they also contribute to the rise in inflammatory diseases.

Our Artificial Environment

The Western lifestyle has led to most people living in an increasingly artificial environment. Three out of four people in Germany are drawn to the emerging urban areas with their attractive offers of jobs, education, and culture. The disadvantages, however, are not to be overlooked: Most people live in cramped apartments, while traffic and industry burden us with exhaust gases, fine dust, and noise. The sensory overload stresses people. Moreover, modern Homo sapiens spend about 90% of their time indoors. Even when you are outdoors, it does not necessarily mean health-promoting contact with nature, because, in the cities, the ground is further sealed with asphalt over large areas. Even on a walk through settlements in urban outskirts, one notices that the labor-saving habit of covering front yard gardens with gravel or stones is becoming more and more prevalent. It may be that a vegetable garden requires too much effort and knowledge, but lack of time and convenience leads to even lawns and flower beds becoming less common.

Even a trip to the areas surrounding cities is sobering: instead of diverse nature, the lush green of meadows and fields has mainly been replaced by monotonous, heavily fertilized monocultures of high-yield fodder grasses, cereals or rapeseed. Instead of nature, one should rather speak of agricultural steppes here, because rich animal and plant life in Central Europe can now almost only be found in nature reserves or in the cemeteries and railway facilities of the big cities. Conventional agriculture is no longer a source of biological diversity: the economic pressure for mass production, to which most farmers are subjected, has led to the death of farms and the flourishing of the agricultural industry. With industrial agriculture, the agricultural landscape has also changed significantly: fields, pastures and orchards with a rich insect and bird fauna have become cleared, industrially managed, monotonous agricultural landscapes in many places.

The pressure for mass production also necessitates the use of agrochemicals, the diverse effects of which are still little researched. Neonicotinoids bring insect life to a standstill, even in the smallest amounts, and the herbicide glyphosate has effects on the living environment, because it damages the populations of bacteria throughout the biosphere. The consequences of the change are becoming visible in the death of insects and the decline of bird species, which are indicators of a much more extensive process: the diversity of life on earth is decreasing at a rapid pace. The German Nature Conservation Association speaks of the greatest extinction of species since the time of the dinosaurs and suspects that around 150 animal and plant species disappear from the globe every day. Various studies in Germany show that, since 1960, the biomass of insects has decreased by more than 80% and, accordingly, the stocks of field birds are in freefall. This loss of diversity continues at the micro level, so that the biodiversity of soil organisms is also declining (Lupatini et al. 2017).

The artificial environment in which we live confronts us with a variety of harmful conditions and toxic substances, but, on the other hand, stimuli that have been part of our lives for millions of years are missing. Under natural conditions, humans form an ecosystem with the hundreds of species of microbes on their skin, on their mucous membranes and in their intestines that regulates their immune system and activates regulatory cycles of health maintenance in the body. The majority of the cohabitants are permanent guests, but, under natural conditions, humans are also constantly exposed to other organisms through their food, untreated drinking water and contact with soil, plants or animals (Fragiadakis et al. 2019). Some settle on or in their new hosts for a shorter or longer time and influence them. Infections, which used to be more common, also stimulate the immune system and train inhibitory regulatory circuits. However, despite this positive side effect, infections are not to be wished for anyone, because the damage they cause is significantly greater than their benefit.

Modern humans lack the supply of harmless environmental microbes because contact with undisturbed nature has decreased. Anyone who has never been in the forest or waded through mud, but only knows air-conditioned houses, offices and shopping centers, lacks an important part of these stimuli that the immune system needs to function correctly. While children used to play outside on the street or in the forest, they now often spend their time in front of the screen. As studies on traditionally operating farms show, children who are exposed to a variety of environmental bacteria have a reduced risk of inflammatory diseases later on (von Mutius 2015, see also, in Chap. 3, the section on the farm effect). This constant contact with harmless bacteria is missing today, so that the diversity of the microbiome has decreased compared to people living close to nature.

The biodiversity of gut bacteria of the few tribes of hunters and gatherers that still exist today is about 60% higher than that of modern humans (Yatsunenko et al. 2012; Clemente et al. 2015). The global trend towards impoverishment of the external ecosystem is thus followed by an equally global trend towards species loss in our internal ecosystem. Both developments are threatening, but are perceived very differently: While the loss of biodiversity in our external environment has been calling people to action for years, the extinction of species in the microbiome has largely gone unnoticed so far.

The Triumph of the Western Diet

A key feature of the Western lifestyle is diet. Its characteristics are industrially produced foods, which are often rich in sugar and other easily digestible carbohydrates, unhealthy fats, and salt. In contrast, they usually contain little fiber. Often, additives such as preservatives, artificial sweeteners, and emulsifiers are used. Typically, the range of food is limited and rich in calories, but poor in fiber. These calorie-rich, easily digestible meals promote certain types of bacteria, but starve others. Food additives can also have harmful effects on the microbiome, as can some medications and antibiotics. The result of the Western diet is a loss of species and a depletion of the gut flora. Occasionally, this shrunken bacterial community is also referred to as the "Western microbiome". The consequences of this loss are only now being understood. How did this development come about?

After the Second World War, many households still had their own gardens, with vegetables and fruit for their own use. In the settlements built for the workers of the ammunition factory in my hometown at the end of the nineteenth century, each house had a piece of land for its own cultivation. Outbuildings allowed for the keeping of chickens, rabbits, and a pig. One could say that small-scale farming for self-sufficiency was practiced. Foods such as bread, milk, flour, pasta, meat, and fish were bought, but mostly not as packaged industrial products, but rather from artisanal production. Even in the 1960s, most cooking was done at home, and few industrially produced products, let alone ready-to-eat meals, were on the table.

As the economy in post-war Germany got going again, food quickly became cheaper. After the lean war years, people were glad to finally be able to eat their fill again, and indulged in hearty home cooking. However, most cooking was still done at home, even though new, tempting achievements soon emerged: The first pizzeria in Germany opened in Würzburg in 1952 and started the triumph of Italian cuisine. The first fast food restaurant of the Wienerwald chain opened in Munich in 1955 and attracted customers with its slogan, "Today the kitchen stays cold, today we're going to the Wienerwald", promising quick enjoyment. It wasn't long before Coca Cola, cornflakes, ketchup, and soft ice cream from the USA began to arrive. The first kebab shop opened in Berlin in the 1970s, according to legend. However, the idea that it was a German invention is a myth, as meat from the kebab skewer was served in bread in Turkey long before. The first McDonald's restaurant opened in Munich in 1971 and ushered in the burger era in Germany. A burger, fries and a cola—today the epitome of unhealthy eating—had the shine of the new (Schlosser 2003).

With the growing integration of women into the labor market in the 1960s, innovations came along that made cooking easier for the housewife. What was bought was not just food, but also time. Canned food and packet soups were the beginning. Refrigerator, freezer and, later, the microwave followed, paving the way for frozen food and ready-to-eat meals. The burgeoning food industry simultaneously changed the profile of food. Food became an industrial product: dishes had to be easy to produce, storable, and affordable. A wide range of food additives were used to facilitate production, improve consistency, and increase shelf life. Today, we know that some of these legally permitted additives, while not toxic, alter the microbiome (examples of this can be found in Chap. 6, "Food"). The industrial production of food also prevailed because it made food increasingly affordable. In 1960, a household in Germany still had to spend about 38% of its income on food, but, by 2019, this share had dropped to just 14% (Statista 2021), about a third of the original value. Over time, more and more households adopted the convenient ready-made and frozen products. The proportion of highly processed foods has been increasing for years—at the expense of home-cooked meals.

Parallel to the increasing pace of the working world, eating habits also changed drastically. In the old Maigret crime novels from the 1960s, the gentleman commissioner quite naturally goes home every day for lunch and: He walks! He goes home, where the freshly cooked lunch is waiting for him. Such conditions have largely disappeared today. Less and less time is planned for the preparation of meals; cooking at home is no longer popular in many circles. On the supermarket shelves, "convenience food" has taken up a dominant place: industrially produced, ready for the table, the microwave or the salad bowl. Many traditional bakeries and butchers have mutated into bake shops or fast food outlets, where a quick lunch "on the go" is taken on the street or standing, usually also from industrially pre-made products. Younger city dwellers in particular like to "order" from delivery services—preferably pizza. The Corona pandemic has greatly accelerated the triumph of fast food.

The result of these changes in the food system? Hard numbers prove that a far greater amount of unhealthy food is being eaten than before the start of the inflammation era. And the portions being eaten are far larger than what is recommended by the medically defined calorie requirement. In combination with the lack of exercise in work and leisure, this calorie-dense, industrial food promotes overweight, worldwide: Already in 2006, the number of overweight people exceeded the number of hungry people in the world (WHO 2020). Overweight is rampant, and spreading, especially in emerging countries. And changes in the microbiome go hand in hand with unhealthy eating and overweight. This trio favors, among other things, inflammatory diseases.

Live Longer, Sick Longer?

Around 1960, newly retired men and women in Germany could expect to have an average of ten more years of life ahead of them. By 2020, this period had grown to about 20 years, double the length! A pension expert explained this to me. His example vividly illustrates the most important change in health over recent decades: People are living longer.

Exact information on this is provided by the Federal Statistical Office under the keyword "life expectancy". This number indicates how long an average person of a certain birth year is likely to live. In the last 150 years, this value has almost doubled; a significant factor was the decline in infectious diseases, such as tuberculosis, pneumonia, and severe diarrheal diseases. While, back then, about half of all deaths in Central Europe were due to infections, today, it is only about 3% (GBD 2017 Mortality and Cause of Death Collaborators 2018). Hygiene measures and the availability of antibiotics and vaccines in the post-war period ensured that child mortality, in particular, fell, with formerly common diseases almost disappearing from the scene.

Even in recent decades, life expectancy has increased again, thanks to better medical care. According to the Federal Statistical Office, women in Germany born in 1980 could expect to live to be 76.3 years old (men: 69.6 years). Girls born in 2020, on the other hand, have an average of 83.4 years (boys: 76.6 years) ahead of them, about 7 years more than the generation born 40 years earlier. However, whether this upward trend will continue is questionable, as stagnation and even declining trends have been observed in the USA and Great Britain for several years (Ho and Hendi 2018; Woolf and Shoemaker 2019).

Intuitively, one associates longer life with good health, because life, after all, requires a certain degree of health. Upon closer inspection, however, this is not the case, as the statistics of health insurance companies clearly show a correlation between aging and the frequency of chronic diseases. Could it be that the increase in inflammatory diseases is simply a consequence of increased life expectancy? According to the equation: "The older you are, the greater the probability of Allergy & Co."? Studies in societies where people reach an extremely high age do not support this assumption. The incidence, i.e., the frequency of new cases, of inflammatory diseases is not determined by age-related wear and tear, but largely by lifestyle.

In this context, it is instructive to look at areas where a particularly larger number of people reach a very high age. When comparing population data, it was noticed that, in certain regions, the so-called "Blue Zones", the proportion of extremely old people is especially high. Incidentally, the term "Blue Zones" came about because researchers, during a discussion about the age of people in Sardinia, marked a particularly interesting area with a blue ballpoint pen. These Blue Zones include a certain area of Sardinia, the island of Okinawa (Japan) and the island of Ikaria in Greece. Residents of these regions frequently reach an age of over 90 years, some even up to 115 years. The common denominator of the lifestyle of the seniors in these regions is a traditionally shaped life in the countryside, with physical work and an active lifestyle lasting into old age. People eat healthily, often with self-produced food, get a lot of exercise and spend a lot of time outdoors. They are integrated into the family or into a village's social structure.

The seniors in these areas impress with their physical and mental fitness into old age. Hardly any of them suffer from chronic diseases (Poulin 2019), and studies show that inflammatory diseases are much less common there than in other areas. A long life does not necessarily have to be accompanied by chronic suffering! Aging itself is not a disease, but the Western lifestyle promotes diseases in old age. The probability of chronic diseases is largely influenced by health-related behavior. How well do you keep your body in shape? Even with a car that has 150,000 km on the clock, maintenance and care make the difference between a good used car and a rust bucket.

The changes in our lifestyle in recent decades are so drastic that one cannot simply beam back to 1960 in the hope of living more healthily. That would not be desirable anyway, because our life today is overall easier, and we have the chance to enjoy it significantly longer than we would have just a few decades ago. The question is rather, how can we benefit from the conveniences of modern life without increasing the risk of chronic diseases? A first important step is to recognize that microbes are an important part of our life and contact with them is essential for our own health. We cannot separate our inner environment from the rest of our lives but must rather steer the balance with it in the right direction. Living longer can thus also mean enjoying one's longer life in good health.

References

ADAC (2010) ADAC Mobilitätsstudie 2010, Munich. https://www.adac.de/_mmm/pdf/statistics_mobility_in_germany_0111_46603.pdf

Clemente JC et al (2015) The microbiome of uncontacted amerindians. Science Adv 1: e1500183

Fragiadakis GK et al (2019) Links between environment, diet, and the hunter-gatherer microbiome. Gut Microbes 10:216–227

GBD 2017 Causes of Death Collaborators (2018) Global, regional, and national age-sex-specific mortality for 282 causes of death in 195 countries and territories, 1980 – 2017: A systematic analysis for the Global Burden of Disease Study 2017. Global Health Metrics 392:1736–1788

Ho J, Hendi A (2018) Recent trends in life expectancy across high income countries: retrospective observational study. BMJ 362:2562

JIM (2019) JIM Study 2019. Jugend, information, Medien. Medienpädagogischer Forschungsverband Südwest. https://www.mpfs.de/fileadmin/files/Studies/JIM/2019/JIM_2019.pdf

Kondrashova A et al (2012) The 'Hygiene hypothesis' and the sharp gradient in the incidence of autoimmune and allergic diseases between Russian Karelia and Finland. Acta Pathol Microbiol Immunol Scand 121:478–493

Krämer U et al (2014) What can reunification of East and West Germany tell us about the cause of the allergy epidemic? Clin Exp Allergy 45:94–107

Lupatini M et al (2017) Soil microbiome is more heterogeneous in organic than in conventional farming system. Front Microbiol 7. https://doi.org/10.3389/fmicb.2016.02064

Poulin M (2019) Individual longevity versus population longevity. In: Caruso C (ed) Centenarians. Springer, Berlin, Heidelberg

Rukolainen L et al (2017) Significant disparities in allergy prevalence and microbiota between the young people in Finnish and Russian Karelia. CEA 47:665–674

Schlosser E (2003) Fast food Gesellschaft: Fette Gewinne, faules system. Riemann-Verlag, Munich

Statista (2021). https://de.statista.com/statistik/daten/studie/75719/mfrage/ausgaben-fuer-nahrungsmittel-in-Deutschland-seit-1900. Accessed 10 Jan 021

TK (2016) Beweg Dich, Deutschland. Bewegungsstudi2 2016. https://www.tk.de/resource/blob/2033598/9f2d920e270b7034df3239cbf1c2a1eb/move-germany-data.pdf

Vatanen T et al (2016) Variation in microbiome LPS immunogenicity contributes to autoimmunity in humans. Cell 165:842–853

Von Mutius E (2015) The microbial environment and its influence on asthma prevention in early life. J Allergy Clin Immunol 137:1–10

Von Mutius E et al (1998) Increasing prevalence of hay fever and atopy among children in Leipzig, East Germany. Lancet 35:862–866

WHO (2020) Obesity and overweight. Fact sheets. https://www.who.int/news-room/fact-sheets/detail/obesity-and-overweight. Accessed 10 Jan 2020

Woolf SH, Shoemaker H (2019) Life expectancy and mortality rates in the United States, 1959—2017. JAMA 322:1996–2016

Yatsunenko T et al (2012) Human gut microbiome viewed across age and geography. Nature 486:222–228

3

From Hygiene to Biodiversity Hypothesis

Contents

Infections as Inflammation Brake: The Hygiene Hypothesis

In England, the increase in allergies and asthma after the Second World War was so strong that it was referred to as the "allergic epidemic" or "post-industrial epidemic". Common roots of allergies, asthma and neurodermatitis were suspected, but the triggers were unknown, and it was assumed that viral infections were the cause. A turning point was the famous publication in 1989 by British epidemiologist David Strachan from the University of London (Strachan 1989). His data suggested that infections, which lead to inflammation in the short term, reduced the frequency of allergies in the long term. Strachan examined the occurrence of hay fever, i.e., an allergy to plant pollen, in over 17,000 children who were born during a certain week in March 1954, and were followed up to the age of 23. Of the 16 points of collected data on birth, social status and environment, two factors showed a clear correlation with hay fever: The larger a family, the less likely the children were to have

© The Author(s), under exclusive license to Springer Nature Switzerland AG 2025
R. Lucius, *The Microbiome*, https://doi.org/10.1007/978-3-031-78821-5_3

allergies to pollen in later life. In addition, children with older siblings were better protected against hay fever than the first-borns. Strachan's unadorned publication takes up less than two printed pages, but has since been cited over 6000 times in scientific publications. In it, he speculated that, as a family grows in size, the younger siblings are exposed to infections that they catch from the older children. He was thinking of pathogens that are transmitted through direct contact or dirt, such as the Hepatitis A virus or the parasite Toxoplasma gondii. Contrary to the prevailing opinion at the time, Strachan suspected that the excessive immune reactions in allergies were not triggered by pathogens, but that infections, on the contrary, provided protection against them.

The bold idea that contacts with viruses, bacteria and parasites, which demonstrably massively stimulate the immune system, should, at the same time, have a braking effect on allergies diametrically contradicted the prevailing dogma. The reactions ranged from head shaking to massive criticism. This connection between pathogens and allergies was too paradoxical! Since Strachan mentioned, in his short article, a transmission of infections through "unhygienic contacts", his assumption was referred to as the "hygiene hypothesis". This term is not exactly optimal, as the transmission of infectious diseases, which Strachan actually addressed, is not solely determined by hygiene behavior. However, it was perhaps this catchy term that helped the idea to break through. But the message of the new hypothesis was much more differentiated, namely: "Infections can protect against allergies in the long term". It turned out that this was essentially correct. It was later found that other types of microbial contact—such as environmental bacteria or the microbiome—also have protective effects, a fact that does not detract from the hygiene hypothesis.

Initially viewed very skeptically in professional circles at the end of the twentieth century, the hygiene hypothesis established itself over time and was substantiated by new facts. For example, it was shown that children who had two or more colds with fever in their first year of life had a reduced asthma risk of about 50% when they were 7 years old (Illi et al. 2001).

Above all, the hygiene hypothesis was compatible with many new observations. Results from the then-burgeoning field of immunology suggested that the reduced frequency of infections in modern societies, thanks to the use of antibiotics and vaccinations, had led to a change in immune responses. Previously, the frequent infections with viruses and bacteria had shaped the human immune system. Such pathogens cause strong inflammatory reactions that must be actively downregulated after the infection subsides. The immune system learns and trains itself in this process of slowing down with each new infection. If this training is omitted with the decline of infections, the ability to suppress irrelevant immune responses also atrophies.

While the hygiene hypothesis was initially based mainly on studies of allergic diseases, further observations were soon added: Increases in the number of cases of autoimmune diseases such as chronic inflammatory bowel diseases, type 1 diabetes, and multiple sclerosis had also been observed in the post-war decades, a fact that could be explained by the decline in infections. Mouse models offered a litmus test for the hygiene hypothesis, and, indeed, it was unequivocally demonstrated that both infections with live pathogens and treatment with extracts or individual components of microbes could inhibit the onset of various inflammatory diseases (Bach 2018). These findings confirmed the idea that infections train regulatory circuits of the immune system, which reduce the tendency towards inflammatory responses.

Parasitic Worms as Sophisticated Immunologists

Among the pathogens with a particularly strong protective effect against inflammatory diseases are parasitic worms. They are not counted as part of the microbiome in the strict sense, because they are much larger than "microbes", i.e., viruses, bacteria, or single-celled organisms. Just like these, worm parasites are inhabitants of humans or animals and use similar strategies to optimally exploit their hosts. These wonders of nature, which, unfortunately, are usually only seen as a manifestation of ugliness, specifically interfere with certain communication processes of the immune system and switch off inflammatory responses. The simple reason: They do not want to be killed by inflammation. The strategies of the bacteria, which we are only now getting to know with the advent of microbiome research, could be very similar, so it is worth taking a closer look at worm parasites.

Most parasitic worms inhabit the intestines of their hosts, but there are also species that live in the skin or directly in the blood. Their size varies from a few millimeters to—believe it or not—20 meters. In modern societies, they are virtually extinct, as the transmission from one host to the next no longer works in the age of flush toilets, washing machines, and vacuum cleaners. However, they are still widespread in developing countries. Most worm parasites exploit their hosts relatively gently in order to be able to use them for many years.

Adapted over millions of years to a life in a living host, they have learned, through evolution, to manipulate the human immune system in every possible way to nip inflammation in the bud. Parasites deceive, trick, and camouflage to avoid being eliminated by inflammatory responses. Only those who could evade, redirect, or deflect the immune response survived. Thus, evolution has made parasites the cleverest of all immunologists. There have always been observations that allergies and autoimmune diseases are rare in people with worm infections, but it was only with the advent of molecular biological methods that the reasons for this were understood.

My prime example of a parasitic worm that incapacitates its host's immune system is the nematode Onchocerca volvulus, the cause of "river blindness" in tropical Africa. Like most other worm parasites, this animal is a long-term strategist. The adult worms live right in the connective tissue of the human subcutaneous layer and can survive up to 15 years. The females are about 50 cm long and half a millimeter thick, but they curl up such that they could fit in a hazelnut. Through mechanisms that are not yet known, they stimulate the host to form connective tissue around them. Thus, they are literally walled in by host cells and lie in a nodule that is usually easily palpable in the skin. Only the front end, where the sexual and birth opening is located, protrudes from this nodule. The Onchocerca males are about 4 cm long and very mobile. They crawl through the connective tissue of the subcutaneous layer, and thus reach the females to fertilize them.

After mating, the Onchocerca female becomes a birthing machine, producing about 1000 larvae a day. These larvae are about 1/3 millimeter long and survive for about a year. Typical Onchocerca patients, however, do not just have one worm, their nodules rather harbor several dozens of females, so that several million larvae can be wriggling in a human's skin (Schulz-Key 1990). The tiny worms crawl around in the top layers of skin and wait to be picked up by a blood-sucking blackfly, which then transmits them to the next human. On their journey, they can also get into the eye, where they cause many people to go blind. Even today, about 20 million people in Africa are still infected (WHO 2018).

Together with colleagues from the University of Yaoundé, my working group in Cameroon investigated how Onchocerca affects the immune system of humans. When you finally see the patients in a small field hospital after a long drive over potholed tracks, you are amazed: The people suffer from itching, skin changes, and eye problems, including blindness. These symptoms are caused by dead larvae. The skin nodules, in which the worms lie, can be felt under the skin, without causing the slightest pain. There are also no signs of inflammation, such as swelling, redness, or warmth. Quite obviously, the Onchocerca females can lie for years as foreign bodies in the skin without being attacked by the immune system. Even the living larvae do not activate the immune system in most people. How can 50 cm-long worms and millions of larvae live in the skin of a human without causing a fulminant inflammation? Every splinter that tears into your flesh causes a painful, suppurating abscess if it is not removed quickly.

When you prepare surgically removed worm nodules, make thin tissue sections of them and stain them, the first impression is confirmed when looking into the microscope: In the dense connective tissue that surrounds the worms, you see no accumulations of inflammatory cells; the nodule is, so to speak, immunologically silent. This is similar to what one sees with the larvae in the skin of most Onchocerca patients: In section preparations, you can see the living mini worms lying directly in the skin, without any signs of inflammation being discernible. However, this is only true as long as the larvae live. If you find dead larvae, you can see inflammatory cells around them that pounce on the parasites and destroy them (Bryceson 1976; Medina-De la Garza et al. 1990). The same also applies to larvae that happen to die in the eye. There, inflammations form around dead parasites, which cloud the cornea and also cause severe destruction in other parts of the eye, sometimes leading to blindness. Obviously, living parasites can stop immune responses, while dead worms are immediately attacked. This raised the question: Do the living worms release substances for their own protection that defuse the immune responses of the human host?

Studies of a related worm parasite that infects rodents offered the solution. We were able to study these nematodes under defined investigating conditions in the lab. It was found that living adult worms and larvae constantly secrete the small protein Cystatin. Onchocerca worms and their larvae also produce this active ingredient. Cystatin is found in many organisms and inhibits certain enzymes within cells. However, the parasitic nematodes have modified the protein over the course of evolution so that it is released externally into the host and alters the function of immune cells (Hartmann and Lucius 2003). Years of studies by my former colleague and current professor of immunology, Susanne Hartmann, revealed an interesting mechanism of action of Cystatin:

When the protein is recognized by phagocytes (macrophages) of the mouse or the human, it initially stimulates an inflammatory reaction, but within a few hours, it reprograms the cells: Originally aggressive, inflammation-promoting macrophages are polarized by the worm protein. They then specifically send signals to further immune cells, which, in turn, release an inflammation-inhibiting messenger substance, the cytokine IL-10. In this way, they block the immune attack and calm the immune system (Ziegler et al. 2015).

Our experiments showed that the anti-inflammatory effect of Cystatin is so strong that, in mice, injections of the worm protein block the development of allergies to grass pollen or chicken protein. Similarly, experiments showed that Cystatin in mice also prevents the development of an intestinal inflammation that corresponds to human ulcerative colitis. Other research groups also showed a similar effect of proteins from other parasitic worms. In experiments with rodents, worm products prevented or slowed down allergies, asthma, colitis, type 1 diabetes, a disease similar to multiple sclerosis, and pneumonia.

Not only does Onchocerca volvulus inhibit inflammatory responses in humans, but many other parasitic worms do as well: They prevent themselves from being destroyed by the immune system, but, at the same time, protect their host against excessive immune responses. Over the course of co-evolution, the human immune system has probably become accustomed to this inflammation brake. It has become used to, so to speak, constantly driving with the brake applied. When this brake is removed, because parasitic worms have virtually become extinct due to modern hygiene, the engine revs too high: The unbraked inflammatory responses manifest themselves in the form of diseases.

Thus, the worms have a positive property, although, in most cases, the health damage they cause outweighs this. Nevertheless, there have been many attempts to use worm parasites to cure inflammatory diseases. Especially in the USA, there is a whole scene of patients who self-treat with parasitic worms, report results on internet forums and exchange worm eggs among each other. If you visit the "Helminthic Therapy Wiki", for example, you enter a medical parallel world in which worm therapy is used for a variety of diseases. In the real world, the success of such treatments seems to be limited to individual cases, so that inflammation inhibitors based on parasites have not yet found their way into clinics.

Although parasitic worms and commensal bacteria are very different organisms, both have very similar interests. Both depend on exploiting their host in the long term and benefit from a restrained immune system, which, on the other hand, allows for an efficient defense against pathogens. Therefore, it is to be expected that the commensals apply similar strategies as the worm parasites and influence the host's immune system in a similar way. So far, little is known about this, because microbiome research is still young, but the prospects for exciting research results are very good.

The Farm Effect: Health from the Cowshed

With the advent of the hygiene hypothesis, protection against inflammatory diseases was initially only attributed to infections, but this view changed when systematic studies investigated the comparative frequency of allergic diseases in urban and rural children. For example, a Swedish study of over 1 million recruits showed that, between 1952 and 1989, the frequency of hay fever, asthma, and eczema had quadrupled (Braback et al. 2004). Urban dwellers were far more likely to be plagued by allergic diseases than rural inhabitants. The Swedish health registers were so meticulously maintained that further highly interesting information could be obtained by additionally distinguishing between rural children and farmer's children: children from farming families were less affected by the diseases than children of forest workers. Apparently, living directly on a farm protected against allergic diseases, but living in the countryside in general did not.

Worldwide, in various European countries, but also in the USA and New Zealand, studies revealed a consistent pattern. Children who had grown up on farms were less likely to suffer from hay fever, asthma, or eczema than city children (von Mutius 2015). A Swedish publication describes that city children have an eight times higher allergy risk compared to farm children (Jonsson et al. 2016). In many of these studies, pediatrician and allergist Erika von Mutius, now director of the Institute for Asthma and Allergy Research at the Helmholtz Center in Munich, was a driving force, constantly breaking new ground. In a famous study, she showed, using the example of the Amish and the Hutterites, two American religious communities, that even the type of farming makes a difference: children of the Amish, who have maintained traditional farming and still use horses and carts today, are more protected against allergic diseases than children of the Hutterites, who practice motorized farming in a modern style (Stein et al. 2016). This example is detailed in the sidebar "Farm and farm are not the same" on the book's website.

In several of these studies, it was found that the frequency of allergic diseases correlated with contact with livestock and pets. In this case, children from dairy farms were notably well protected.

Interestingly, this protection was partly due to the consumption of raw milk, as later studies revealed, while pasteurized milk had no effect. This protective effect is partly due to heat-labile components of the milk, the identification of which is now being worked on. Also, the presence of dogs in the household had a positive effect but contact with several types of animals also provided stronger protection than with just one type of animal. Even though the protective "farm effect" was mainly worked out using the example of allergic diseases, it was not limited to them. The likelihood of later suffering from chronic intestinal inflammation was also reduced in children from farming families (Radon et al. 2007).

In large-scale studies, it was also found that protection against allergic diseases was most pronounced when children were exposed to the rural environment in the womb and during the first year of life (Smits et al. 2016). The first 100 days of life were particularly important (Stiemsma and Turvey 2017). Under farm conditions, the risk of developing asthma later was reduced by about 25%, while the risk of hay fever and eczema was as much as halved (von Mutius 2015). This particular effectiveness of the farm effect in early childhood shows, like other research results, that a long-term programming of the still immature child's immune system takes place during this period. Early contact with the farm environment leads to later immune tolerance!

The effect of protection against allergic diseases lasted the longest if the children continued to live on the farm. If children who had grown up on a farm later moved to the city, the protective effect decreased over time. How long the protective effect of rural life lasts is shown by a Polish study comparing the frequency of allergies before and after Poland's entry into the European Union: Within just 9 years after joining the EU, the number of allergic diseases among the Polish rural population had almost doubled due to changes in living conditions (Sozanska et al. 2014). The Western lifestyle had boosted Allergies & Co. within a few years!

The farm children offered a chance to make progress in the search for the mysterious key factors that affect the immune system. Bacteria ultimately turned out to be a decisive factor that reduced the inflammatory reactions of farm children, occurring in great diversity in the environment and not causing infections. On the examined farms, such bacteria were found in large quantities, for example, in old-fashioned cowsheds (Ege 2017). Where hay and beets are fed to the animals, remnants of manure lie around, flies buzz, and swallows crisscross the air, one will find a diverse and dense bacterial flora and many other microbes. One rich source for bacteria was dust, which is also brought into the home of farmers from the cattle shed. In addition to living bacteria, it also contains many bacterial components, including substances that strongly activate the immune system. However, this mixture also trains inhibitory immune mechanisms and causes immune tolerance in a similar way to infectious agents.

This highly effective dust is inhaled, swallowed, and absorbed through skin wounds. The ways in which it can affect the immune system can be seen in, among other things, studies in animal models: If you let mice inhale dust from homes of farming families who practice dairy farming in traditional, old-fashioned style, allergic reactions are suppressed. In contrast, the dust from households of modern farmers intensified allergies in the animals. Analyses showed that individual bacterial species from the dust were particularly efficient at inhibiting immune responses, such as Acinetobacter lwoffi and Lactobacillus iners. However, the best damping effect was achieved by a mixture of as many species as possible (Ober et al. 2017). In the same vein, there are also studies that examine the relationship between dust from homes and the asthma risk of the residents (Kirjavainen et al. 2019; Karvonen et al. 2019). Many more bacteria that came from the environment and from animals were found in the dust from the homes of children who were not affected by asthma than in the dust of the homes of asthmatic children. These observations found their reflection in the "biodiversity hypothesis" (Haahtela 2019). It states that a broad spectrum of bacterial stimuli is optimal to induce immune tolerance.

So, will there be a "cowshed as nasal spray" product in the pharmacy around the corner in the future? Probiotic bacteria to inhale? Before it comes to that, there would still be some questions to clarify: The most important would be the one about the bacteria species used. Given the strict requirements for the safety of medicines, bacteria species that could cause diseases in people with weakened immune systems would certainly be ruled out from the start. An example of this is Acinetobacter, a genus of bacteria that are widely spread in soils, water and wastewater. They seem to mediate immune tolerance, but, in hospitals and care facilities, they appear as opportunistic (i.e., pathogenic for susceptible patients) pathogens. The question would also be whether a brief contact with the effective, tolerance-inducing microbes is sufficient. Would one inhalation per day be enough, or would one have to be exposed to the bacteria permanently? And: Would such a bacterial therapy only have a preventive effect or could it also be used for the treatment of already established diseases, making the application much more attractive? Clearly, a lot of research is still needed.

References

Bach JF (2018) The hygiene hypothesis in autoimmunity: the role of pathogens and commensals. Nat Rev Immunol 18:105–121

Braback L et al (2004) Trends in asthma, allergic rhinitis and eczema among Swedish conscripts from farming and non-farming environments. A nationwide study over three decades. Clin Exp Allergy 34:38–43

Bryceson AD (1976) What happens when microfilariae die? Trans Roy Soc Trop Med Hyg 70:397–401

Ege MJ (2017) The hygiene hypothesis in the age of the microbiome. Ann Am Thorac Soc 14(suppl. 5):348–353

Haahtela T (2019) A biodiversity hypothesis. Allergy 2019:1–12

Hartmann S, Lucius R (2003) Modulation of host immune responses by nematode cystatins. Int J Parasitol 33:1291–1302

Illi S et al (2001) Early childhood infectious diseases and the development of asthma up to school age: a birth cohort study. BMJ 322:390–395

Jonsson K et al (2016) Fat intake and breast milk fatty acid composition in farming and nonfarming women and allergy development in the offspring. Pediatr Res 79:114–123

Karvonen A et al (2019) Indoor bacterial microbiota and development of asthma by 10.5 years of age. J Allergy Clin Immunol S 144(19):31033–31034

Kirjavainen PV et al (2019) Farm-like indoor microbiota in non-farm homes protects children from asthma development. Nat Med 25:1089–1095

Medina-De la Garza CE et al (1990) Serum-dependent interaction of granulocytes with Onchocerca volvulus microfilariae in generalized and chronic hyper-reactive onchocerciasis and its modulation by diethylcarbamazine. Trans R Soc Med Hyg 84:701–706

Ober C et al (2017) Immune development and environment: lessons from Amish and Hutterite children. Curr Opin Immunol 48:51–60

Radon K et al (2007) Contact with farm animals in early life and juvenile inflammatory bowel disease: a case-control study. Pediatrics 120:354–361

Schulz-Key H (1990) Observations on the reproductive biology of Onchocerca volvulus. Acta Leiden 59:27–44

Smits HH et al (2016) Childhood allergies and asthma: new insights on environmental exposures and local immunity at the lung barrier. Curr Opin Immunol 42:41–47

Sozanska B et al (2014) Atopy and allergic respiratory disease in rural Poland before and after accession to the European Union. J Allergy Clin Immunol 133:1347–1353

Stein MM et al (2016) Innate immunity and asthma risk in Amish and Hutterite farm children. N Engl J Med 375:411–421

Stiemsma LT, Turvey E (2017) Asthma and the microbiome: defining the critical window in early life. Allergy Asthma Clin Immunol 13:3

Strachan DP (1989) Hay fever, hygiene and household size. BMJ 299:1259–1260

Von Mutius E (2015) The microbial environment and its influence on asthma prevention in early life. J Allergy Clin Immunol 137:1–10

WHO (2018) Onchocerciasis. Available: https://www.who.int/news-room/factsheets/detail/onchocerciasis. Accessed 30 Jan 2020

Ziegler T et al (2015) A novel regulatory macrophage induced by a helminth molecule instructs Il-10 in CD4+ cells and protects against mucosal inflammation. J Immunol 194:1555–1564

4

Humans and the Microbiome: We Are Many

Contents

The Microbiome: More Than Just a Fad

While science focused on infectious pathogens and environmental bacteria as triggers of the inflammation brake, the microbiome remained an unknown quantity for a long time. Only when the new techniques of high-throughput sequencing of DNA became available from the 2010s onwards did researchers throw themselves into this white spot on the map and analyze the bacterial flora of even the most remote corner of the body. It became clear that the microbiome of the gut, mucous membranes, and skin was another important group of bacteria influencing the immune system. The infectious pathogens and environmental bacteria did not lose their importance, but they did take a back seat for a while; their research is only now being reactivated—rather tentatively. The star, the "new girl in town", is now the microbiome.

The reasons for the attractiveness of the microbiome as a research area are obvious: Due to their massive number, the bacteria of the microbiome, which are in constant close contact with the body, have the potential to significantly shape humans. In terms of numbers alone, the bacteria of the large intestine are the most significant, as they make up 99% of the total microbiome. The majority of our gut flora consists of peaceful bacteria that provide various services in exchange for food and warmth, such as the supply of energy and metabolic products. Another service that we seem to have outsourced to the microbiome over the course of evolution is the regulation of inflammatory responses. Apparently, there has been a certain division of labor: The bulk of immune regulation is done by the body itself, ensuring that dangerous foreign substances are recognized and attacked, while components of the actual body are spared. However, when it comes to slowing down inflammation, we seem to have given the microbes a say and, in this way, ensured that immune responses to irrelevant stimuli are scaled down appropriately.

One might wonder if microbiome research is just a fad that will soon be overtaken by the next trend. This is rather unlikely, as viewing humans as a superorganism, which forms a functional unit with its inhabitants and its living environment, opens up many new opportunities for the prevention and cure of diseases. The aspect that the microbiome can easily be influenced by diet or medication, allowing one to control the species composition, is very attractive. The bacterial flora can also be changed in a desired direction through contact with nature, targeted intake of probiotics, or exercise. Start-ups are already developing bacterial mixtures to get the gut of patients back on track after antibiotic or chemotherapy. If, in a few years, the role of the individual bacterial species of the microbiome and their cooperation as an ecosystem is better known, it will certainly be possible to put together individually adapted microbiomes that harmonize optimally with the respective human being. And, last but not least, tailor-made bacteria of the microbiome could equip their host with additional, useful properties, for example, to tap into other food sources, produce vitamins, or balance the immune system. However, in relation to inflammatory diseases, one should not forget that, despite the current focus on the microbiome, infectious pathogens and environmental microbes also significantly influence the immune system.

The Human as a Superorganism

Even the first humans must have been aware that they were colonized from both outside and inside. After all, lice, fleas, and mites belong to the completely natural fauna of humans, not to mention blood-sucking short-term visitors like mosquitoes, ticks and horseflies. However, intestinal parasites, which are occasionally excreted with the stool, are also noticeable. Roundworms of about 20 cm in length, but also smaller worms or tapeworm segments, which can move noticeably, are hard to overlook and have always aroused the interest of physicians. In the Egyptian Papyrus Ebers from the sixteenth century BC, one of the oldest medical texts, these intestinal parasites are already described, and remedies and magical formulas for their combat are listed. For quite a long time, the parasitic worms, which could be studied with the naked eye or simple microscopes, remained the only known pathogens.

Bacteria only entered the world stage in 1675, when the Dutchman Antoni van Leeuwenhoek, using his self-built microscopes, saw bacteria that came from his dental plaque. The highly respected cloth merchant and chamberlain of the Dutch city of Delft was a fanatical microscope hobbyist and brought the art of grinding glass lenses to an unprecedented perfection. Initially, bacteria were thought to be small plants (hence the term "flora"), and interest in the tiny creatures was rather academic until the work of Robert Koch, Louis Pasteur and their students in the second half of the nineteenth century burned the horror of bacterial infectious agents into public consciousness. Since then, bacteria have been intuitively associated with disease—and avoided wherever possible. Without a doubt, the work of the great bacteriologists was a blessing, as hygiene, vaccinations and antibiotics pushed back infectious diseases in highly developed countries. It is to this that we owe a drastic reduction in child mortality, and thus a large part of the enormous increase in average life expectancy.

Meanwhile, the attitude towards our inhabitants is changing again, and we recognize that the microorganisms found in healthy humans on skin and mucous membranes, in the intestine and in the lungs complement our organism. Most of these inhabitants have a positive effect. It has been known for some time that intestinal bacteria produce such vital substances as vitamins B12, B2 and K, as well as folic acid and biotin. This function is often considered the most important aspect of the coexistence of humans and bacteria. However, we get most vitamins directly from food, because hardly any vitamins are absorbed from the large intestine, where the majority of bacteria live. In addition, our intestinal inhabitants also contribute certain amino acids, which humans can only produce to a limited extent.

It should also be mentioned that some intestinal bacteria can produce extremely harmful substances. An example is trimethylamine, which is produced by certain bacteria from carnitine, a component of red meat (Koeth et al. 2019). More information on this can be found in the "Macro and Micronutrients" section in Chap. 8.

The importance of bacteria as vitamin producers is undisputed, but much more important is their role as protectors against pathogens and educators of the immune system. After all, humans could quickly be overrun by harmful bacteria if their surfaces were not densely populated with commensal bacteria that defend their territories against intruders. The local inhabitants not only occupy the docking sites and consume the available nutrients, but also drive away strangers with sophisticated antibacterial molecules. In particular, the intestine, which is predestined as an entry point for pathogens, is thus kept free of invaders in cooperation with the immune system.

This immune system does have potent defense mechanisms but can only use them in moderation. Only a well-balanced immune system ensures that, on the one hand, pathogens are attacked, but, on the other hand, the body itself is spared, along with beneficial bacteria. Especially in the early childhood phase, the inhabitants of the intestine, skin and mucous membranes program the response of the immune system, and thus determine how the body reacts to stimuli later in life (discussed in detail in the section "The long-term programming of immune tolerance" in this chapter).

For many people, it takes a little getting used to the idea, but we form a community together with bacteria, archaea (primitive single cells), viruses, parasites and fungi, which frolic on or in us from childhood. One is tempted to speak of humans as a living zoo, but that does not really hit the factual mark. We are more than that: We form a community with the microbes that bustle on and in us, with the "microbiome", a community of life for mutual profit, a close partnership. Humans and microbes together form a "superorganism".

According to estimates, about 10,000 different species of bacteria live on and in humans worldwide (Pasolli et al. 2019; for the concept of species in bacteria, see the excursion "Bacteria and the concept of species" in Chap. 8). Even if this estimate turns out to be high, the diversity is enormous. How close this coexistence is and how far humans and their peaceful inhabitants, the commensal bacteria, have engaged in evolution has only become clear in recent years.

What would happen if we had no inhabitants? No one can answer this question, because there are probably no humans without a microbiome. However, the consequences of a life without microbes can be simulated in mice: If you let the rodents grow up completely sterile, some organs and certain behaviors develop differently. To effect this, baby mice are delivered by caesarean section, kept in a sterile environment and supplied with sterilized food and filtered air. Under these conditions, the intestine of the animals is completely free of bacteria. In such mice, the liver is not fully developed, the appendix is huge, and the immune system does not function properly. Because hardly any antibodies are formed, the number of immune cells is reduced to about half and no memory cells are formed; the animals become highly sensitive to infections. Even if they get the same food as animals with an intestinal flora, they form up to 40% less fat than normal animals. In addition, it is striking that sterile mice also have a less pronounced memory for spatial conditions, are more anxious and much more susceptible to stress, and interact less with other mice. If the animals are then colonized with intestinal bacteria, these deficits can be partially reversed. It is clear: bacteria are not just random inhabitants or pathogens in mice. Without them, the mouse is not complete.

But can germ-free mice also survive in the long term and reproduce? Uli Steinhoff, Professor of Immunology and Microbiology at the University of

Marburg, has been researching the connection between microbiome and immune response for more than 20 years. He reassures me: Mice get through life very well without a microbiome, with good nutrition and reproduction works, as long as they are isolated from the environment, i.e., do not come into contact with pathogens. They even have advantages compared to normal animals: Because' they have a less active metabolism and are slimmer, they live a few weeks longer than animals with a normal intestinal flora (Tazume et al. 1991). Transferred to humans, this would mean a gain of a few years. The big disadvantage, however, is that even a few harmful bacteria can lead to deadly infections in sterile mice, while animals with a microbiome only get sick with much larger infection doses (Mittrücker et al. 2016). The intestinal bacteria thus make it difficult for pathogens to colonize the intestine, because they cause "colonization resistance".

The peaceful bacteria in the gut are therefore health promoters: A colonization with bacteria contributes to the development of the body, keeps pathogens at bay and helps to digest food. Moreover, we know today that the microbiome is also extraordinarily important for the shaping and balance of the immune system. This is not only true for mice, but also for humans. Our beneficial inhabitants are therefore a vital part of our superorganism. Nowadays, it is even a consideration as to which bacteria astronauts should definitely have with them on longer journeys into space in order to stay healthy (Saeei and Barzegari 2012)! So, if humans ever colonize Mars, they would do well not to forget their friends, because, without them, our organism does not function properly—and not just on Mars.

Bacteria: Once Yuck, Now Yay

The bacterial flora of humans has long led a scientific niche existence, and its importance was incredibly underestimated. Although it has been known for many decades that the intestinal tract of animals teems with living organisms, this inner ecosystem has been largely ignored. For a long time, it was even suspected that the large intestine, where the majority of bacteria are located, was a kind of waste bin. Through toxins, the intestinal inhabitants would cause many ailments, including mental illnesses such as depression and schizophrenia. As late as 1900, Nobel laureate Ilya Ilyich Mechnikov, a significant immunologist, theorized that the large intestine of mammals was basically useless. It was only as large as it was so that they could run long distances when fleeing from enemies without having to stop to defecate.

Until the 2000s, there were hardly any bacteria of interest to medical microbiologists other than pathogens, which were to be combated by vaccinations, antibiotics and disinfectants. Until a few years ago, if you wanted to work with commensals, you had to focus on bacteria that could be cultivated with relatively simple methods in the lab. One of many obstacles was the sensitivity of most gut bacteria to atmospheric oxygen, which is only present in minimal concentration in the intestinal lumen. Until recently, only about 30% of the known bacterial species could be cultured, the other approximately 70% being referred to as "dark matter". It was suspected that there must be something important, but there was hardly any progress in getting closer to the matter.

Interest in the topic of the microbiome has changed dramatically since around 2010, when new high-throughput DNA sequencing techniques came on the market, allowing for large-scale sequence analyses to be conducted quickly, and thus very cost-effectively. By determining DNA sequences with "next generation sequencing" (= NGS), it was possible to determine which bacterial species live in and on us. It quickly became clear that our bacterial flora is not only diverse, its composition is also a very personal matter: each person has a flora typical for them, individually different like a fingerprint. Certain vague disease-typical patterns were also observed, suggesting a connection between disturbed bacterial flora and diseases.

For a DNA sequence analysis, as is done in species determination, you need—in short—a biological sample, for example, saliva, tissue or feces, from which you extract DNA. Even from the smallest amounts, DNA can then be amplified using the polymerase chain reaction, and its base sequence is determined by highly sensitive sequencing machines. A gene that is present in all bacteria, the gene for 16S ribosomal RNA, is used as a marker. "16S", in this context, is a size designation for particles. Ribosomes are the protein factories of the cell, linking amino acids to protein chains. They consist largely of RNA, the substance that is otherwise used in the cell as a messenger.

The sequence of the gene that codes for 16S ribosomal RNA is specific to each bacterial species and allows—like a barcode on a product label—for a clear taxonomic assignment. The determined sequences are compared with databases in automated processes. If, for example, the laboratory finds that the 16S rRNA of Ruminococcus bromii was found in a stool sample, the doctor knows that this benign bacterium is part of the patient's intestinal flora. In addition, the amount of DNA found can also provide information about the number of bacteria present. Thanks to the reduced costs, DNA sequencing is now commonplace in research and has also become part of routine diagnostics since the coronavirus pandemic at the latest.

When the enormous possibilities of modern sequencing techniques became clear, the National Health Institute of the USA launched a large research program, the "Human Microbiome Program", into which 940 million dollars flowed over 10 years. For the program, bacterial samples were collected from 300 people from 15 body sites each. From 2007 to 2016, 200 working groups at 80 universities and research institutes sequenced the samples, processed the data, and interpreted them to create a kind of atlas of human bacteria. This program yielded many results and, at the same time, gave research a huge boost through the development of new techniques. However, the program did not fulfill the hope of finding the cause of diseases in a simple way with the intestinal flora. The situation was more complex, but the techniques now available had opened a door. The research community jumped on the new topic, and the emerging hype can certainly be compared with the mood that prevailed when the scope of antibiotics became clear. The major scientific journals are constantly publishing new, exciting findings. Suddenly, researching the once disreputable bacterial flora could build a scientific career!

40 Trillion Inhabitants

On all our surfaces that border the outside world, i.e., on the skin, in the mouth and nose, in the lungs, in the digestive and genital tract, biologists quickly find inhabitants when they search with sensitive methods. Most of the information available concerns bacteria, a fact that corresponds to their great importance as commensals and pathogens. The numbers on the bacteria in the microbiome are truly impressive. In the intestine alone, there are about 40 trillion (not "million" or "billion", but "trillion"!) individual bacteria. In every child, every woman, and every man, there are far more bacteria than there have ever been people living on earth. The vast majority are useful inhabitants who have proven themselves as companions over hundreds of thousands of years, because they provide benefits to their host. But, of course, among the many friendly inhabitants, there are also cheaters who only reap benefits without providing a service in return. As a whole, this bacterial community benefits its host, and it is often difficult to decide to what extent individual species are more commensals or symbionts.

The intestinal bacteria in an average person can weigh about one kilogram. This makes them not quite as heavy as the human brain. But other figures can also be correct, as the amount of intestinal content can vary greatly from person to person. However, these data are only an approximation anyway, as the number of bacteria can change drastically with just one trip to the toilet. If you take the total number of human cells as a basis for calculation, including red blood cells (which do not have a cell nucleus, and are therefore sometimes not counted), the number of bacteria exceeds the number of body cells by about 30% (Sender et al. 2016).

Just as impressive as the bacteria under natural conditions are the parasitic worms, which can compete with bacteria in terms of biomass and have a great influence on the immune system and metabolism of their hosts. There are about 25 species of worm parasites that live of human intestinal content or mucus, and thus usually cause damage to their hosts. Due to their size, worm parasites cannot really be counted as part of the "micro" biome in the strict sense. However, because of their pronounced ability to dampen inflammatory responses, they should not be completely omitted from this book. In Western countries, these interesting inhabitants of humans have almost become extinct due to strict hygiene and flush toilets.

Many viruses are also inhabitants of the intestine. The estimates about the diversity of species vary widely, and it could be that, in the intestine, there are several thousand types of viruses. Most are bacteriophages, i.e., viruses that infect bacteria. Their role in the ecosystem of the intestine is still unclear, but they could contribute to keeping certain bacterial species in check, thus maintaining a balance between the species. A much smaller number of virus species, such as noroviruses, infect the intestinal cells of the host and can cause severe diarrheal diseases. The intestinal flora also includes over a hundred species of lower fungi, which lead an inconspicuous existence under normal circumstances. Archaea, primitive single-celled organisms without a true nucleus, also occur in the intestine.

The estimates of how many bacterial species occur in and on a single average human vary widely; realistically, it should be up to 1000. The greatest diversity is found in the intestine. The spectrum of species present and their proportions vary greatly from person to person, depending on personal history, diet, and lifestyle. The bacterial community of the oral cavity is also very diverse. Other areas, such as the skin, do not offer microorganisms particularly attractive conditions, and are therefore less densely populated, but even there, about 100,000 bacteria can be found per square centimeter, while internal organs are normally germ-free.

A portion of the numerous subtenants is common to many, but not all people: In one study, 57 bacterial species were found in 90% of the subjects (Arumugam et al. 2011). So, there seems to be a core set of species that are, so to speak, the standard inhabitants of humans.

The multitude of bacterial species is indeed astonishing, but even more important is the diversity of metabolic processes that take place in them. Each of these bacteria can be seen as a miniature factory that processes raw materials and generates energy from them as material for operation and reproduction. In addition, metabolic waste products, or "metabolites", are released into the environment. These processes are controlled by genes. Assuming that each bacterial species has about 4000 genes, then the entire bacterial community of a human, with a number of 1000 species, would have a genome of 4000,000 genes—compared to the mere 22,000 genes of humans, an overwhelmingly high number. Thus, over 99% of the genes of the human superorganism are provided by bacteria! However, many of these genes are very similar in different bacteria, a fact that reduces the diversity again. Nevertheless, our bacteria can carry out many more and completely different processes, and thus metabolize other substances that humans cannot. For example, the bacteria of the large intestine probably have about 200 times more enzymes for the breakdown of food residues that are indigestible for us. This explains, for example, the impressive ability of our inhabitants to recycle waste, even breaking down the toughest plant fibers.

Each person has his or her own personal combination of bacteria, which is largely determined by his or her environment and only to a small extent by his or her genetic makeup. A numbers game shows that there is an incomprehensible variety of intestinal floras when you consider all possible combinations of bacterial species and concentrations. Let's assume that, in the intestine of a human, 200 various species of bacteria occur (in reality, the number is probably closer to 1000 species!), with a total of 40 trillion organisms. Theoretically, the number of individuals of each bacterial species can range between a single bacterium and 40 trillion, meaning there are 40 trillion possible different concentrations for each species. If you combine each concentration with each bacterial species, in our example with 200, you get a huge number. The exact calculation of the result is so complex that it is better to estimate the value using a mathematical model. Then, the result, calculated by a friend who is a mathematics professor, is: "about 1.6×10 to the power of 2334". This number would correspond to approximately a 16 followed by 2333 zeros and would take up about three-quarters of a page of this book. That's how low the probability is that two people have exactly the same composition of gut flora! Even if our number game is theoretical, it shows that, given the enormous magnitude of possible combinations on earth, throughout the entire course of human history, there have probably never been two people with identical gut flora.

A Brief Introduction to Bacteria

If you analyze the DNA from different body regions, you mainly find bacterial DNA sequences, in addition to human genetic material. In the gut, usually over 99% of the non-human DNA comes from bacteria, the other 0.9% from viruses, fungi, parasites, and archaea. According to current research, bacteria probably have the greatest influence on humans, so this chapter mainly deals with them. Therefore, here is a brief primer on bacteria:

Bacteria consist of a single cell that does not have a nucleus. This cell is delimited from the outside by a membrane, onto which a highly complex cell wall is superimposed (Fig. 4.1). This surface is special: it consists largely of substances that do not occur in humans and are therefore very well recognized by the immune system.

The immune system detects bacteria as potential pathogens and has developed special sensors to recognize their molecular "trademarks" as danger signals. To defend against them, it immediately triggers a severe inflammation. However, many bacteria have further developed the components of their cell wall so that they no longer stimulate human immune cells particularly strongly or even calm them down. Based on the structure of this cell wall, we distinguish between "gram-positive" bacteria, which can be stained with the Gram stain, and "gram-negative" bacteria, which cannot be stained with it. The bacterial cell wall is constantly being remodeled, so gut bacteria continuously release material, and can thus influence the host (Turroni et al. 2014).

Escherichia Coli: A VIP Among Bacteria

The best-known bacterium is E. coli, an intestinal inhabitant that, however, only makes up about 0.1% of the total bacterial mass in adults. E. coli is—unlike many other bacteria—not sensitive to atmospheric oxygen and can therefore be easily cultivated on agar plates or in simple nutrient solutions. This has made E. coli probably the best-studied organism worldwide and the favorite toy and workhorse of molecular biologists.

Fortunately, E. coli is quite suitable for comparison with many other bacteria. The E. coli cell is rod-shaped, spans 2–6 micrometers (thousandths of a millimeter) and divides in the lab under good growth conditions into two daughter cells within 20 min; in other words, it multiplies very quickly. The same process in the intestine takes much longer. Its elastic cell wall consists of, among other things, lipopolysaccharide (LPS) molecules, which are typical for bacterial surfaces, and thus very strong danger signals for the immune

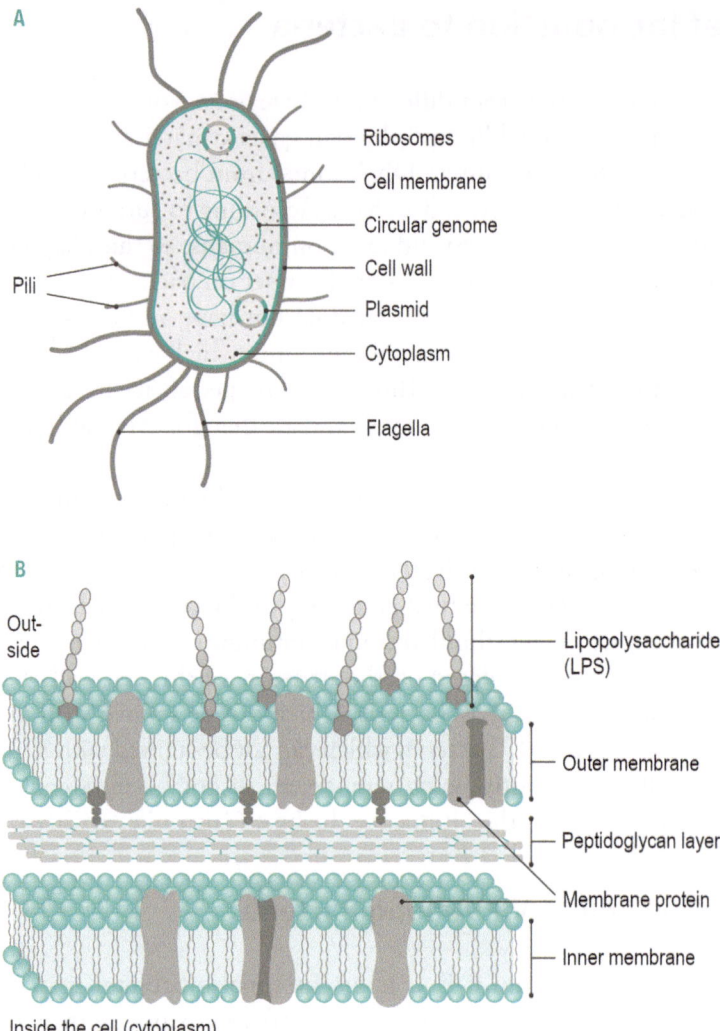

Fig. 4.1 Escherichia coli as an example of the structure of bacteria. (**a**) Organization of the cell. The circular genome lies freely in the cell. E. coli can move with flagella and attaches itself to intestinal cells with pili. (**b**) E. coli is surrounded by a complex cell wall, the components of which (especially LPS) stimulate the immune system. Compiled from various sources. (© Scorpio Verlag in Europa Verlage GmbH, München. Reproduced with permission)

system. Sudden contact with LPS from E. coli and related bacteria has an effect on the immune system like a red rag does to a bull.

E. coli can move using flagella and attach to mucus and cells with thread-like structures. Most strains of E. coli live as commensal bacteria in the intestine. Some strains have taken up genes from other bacteria and can thus cause diseases thanks to new properties. As a result, they can then produce, for example, toxins or can attach particularly well to cells or penetrate them. In this case, they are referred to as pathogenic strains. Other strains of E. coli can have health-promoting effects and are marketed as a "probiotic" (pro = for, bios = life), i.e., a health-promoting preparation. Similarly, strains with very different effects also exist for many other types of bacteria.

The Most Important Bacterial Groups of the Human Microbiome

There is probably no habitat on the globe that is not inhabited by bacteria. The number of recorded species in all biotopes, from the deep sea to the high mountains, is likely to be over 1 million (Louca et al. 2019), although other estimates are much higher. The number of bacterial species on the skin, mucous membranes, in the intestine and in other biotopes of all humanity is estimated to be about 10,000 in total (Pasolli et al. 2019). As already mentioned, a single human hosts up to 1000 species. There are a few dozen core species that occur in most people and very many rare species beyond those (Fig. 4.2). In addition, there are those that enter the intestine with food, drinking water, or in other ways, can hold on for a while and then die out again.

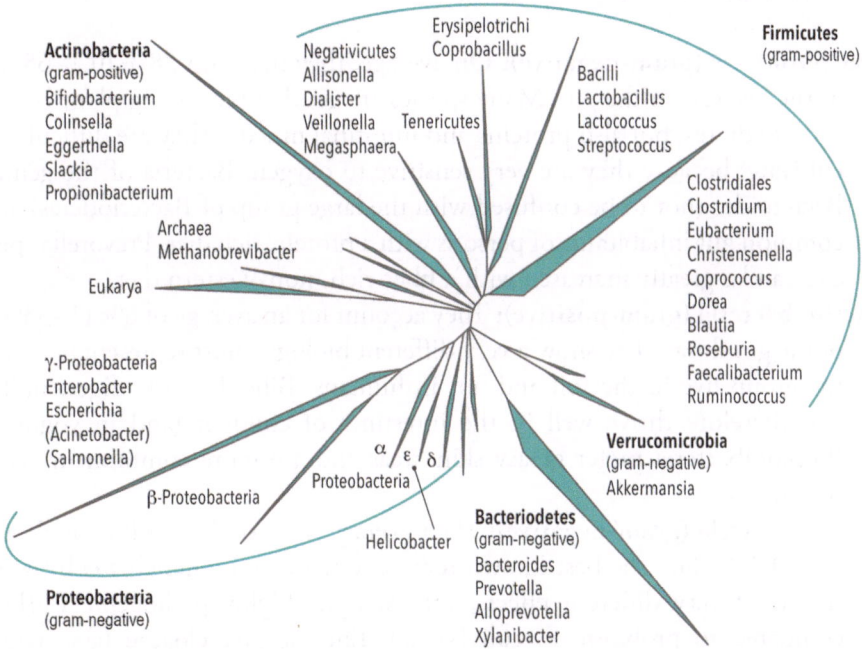

Fig. 4.2 Phylogenetic tree of the most common human gut bacteria. With a Western lifestyle, Firmicutes usually predominate in human microbiomes; with a natural lifestyle, Bacteroidetes are dominant. (Source: Rajilic-Stojanovic et al. 2015. © Scorpio Verlag in Europa Verlage GmbH, München. Reproduced with permission)

In remote regions of Africa and South America, you will find, in addition to the worldwide standard bacteria, certain species that are specifically adapted to the local people. It is also noticeable that, in people living close to nature in such remote areas, the internal species diversity is about 60% greater than in average people from industrialized countries. This imbalance shows that the modern, western lifestyle has led to an "inner species extinction". A world atlas of the peaceful inhabitants of humans would therefore predominantly show a depleted bacterial landscape, and only in a few exotic corners would people in remote areas still have a natural, diverse bacterial flora.

The vast majority of bacterial species of the human microbiome fall within the two very species-rich major groups (scientifically: "Phyla") Firmicutes and Bacteroidetes, as well as the smaller major groups Actinobacteria and Proteobacteria. In total, bacteria of these four major groups make up about 90% of a person's species. Within the major groups, the biology is very different. Among the Proteobacteria are some pathogens, with others that are at least considered harmful and inflammatory. However, they train the immune system, and thus have important functions. Beyond that, one cannot generally assign certain properties to the major groups.

Here are the profiles of the most important bacterial groups and some of their prominent representatives, with quantities referring to people with a "Western lifestyle" (based on Zeißig 2016):

Bacteroidetes (gram-negative): On average, they make up 28% (0.1–65%) of the bacteria in the gut. Many species are good at processing plant-based carbohydrates, but also proteins and intestinal mucus. They are difficult to cultivate, because they are very sensitive to oxygen. Bacteria of the genus Bacteroides (not to be confused with the large group of Bacteriodetes) are common gut inhabitants of persons with a protein-rich diet. Prevotella species can be greatly increased with a fiber-rich, non-Western diet.

Actinobacteria (gram-positive): They account for an average of 8% (1–33%) of the gut flora. They show a very different biology; most representatives of the group live in the soil and not in humans. Bifidobacteria digest milk, and therefore thrive well in the intestines of children (and in yogurt). Propionibacteria prefer greasy skin areas and are more common in acne patients.

Proteobacteria (gram-negative): Their average share of the gut flora is about 2% (0.2–22%). The best-known representatives are Escherichia coli (with strains of very different effects, for example, highly pathogenic EHEC compared to probiotic E. coli Nissle), Enterobacter cloacae (associated with obesity), Helicobacter pylori (potential cause of stomach ulcers) and

Acinetobacter (part of the normal skin flora, but a pathogen in immuno-compromised individuals).

Firmicutes (gram-positive): On average, they make up 39% (20–66%) of the bacterial mass in the intestine and are the most species-rich major group in industrial societies. They usually form quite stable populations. Some can form spores, and therefore spread well. Good processors of simple carbohydrates; have been associated with obesity and Type 2 diabetes. Known representatives are Lactobacillus and Lactococcus (on plants, but also in milk and yogurt), Ruminococcus, the Clostridium species (including C. difficile, a pathogen of potentially fatal diarrheal diseases), Streptococcus (some species of this genus are pathogens, others are commensals), Dorea, Blautia, Roseburia, Faecalibacterium prausnitzii, and Christensenella.

In addition to these important major groups, Akkermansia muciniphila is also worth mentioning as an important bacterium, a species that belongs to the **Verrucomicrobiales**, lives on the mucus layer of the intestine, and can have health-promoting effects.

Some bacterial species are often mentioned in connection with gut health, such as in nutrition studies (Wagenaar et al. 2021). Representatives of these "good" gut inhabitants are, for example, Faecalibacterium prausnitzii, Eubacterium, Bifidobacterium, Roseburia, Lactobacillus, and Akkermansia. However, it must be noted that the effect of bacteria depends very much on the community of microorganisms in which they are embedded. In addition, there are numerous strains of most bacterial species, sometimes with very different properties. Therefore, a blanket statement about the qualities based solely on classification as a species is not possible.

Our Microbial Ecosystem

Like a Forest

If you let the landscape pass by on a train ride in summer, you don't see the individual trees of the forests, but mainly perceive the calming, green tones. It's not for nothing that humans can distinguish more different shades of green than of any other color.

Only on foot do you see the big differences between one forest and another. All forests are complex ecosystems with a variety of trees, shrubs, herbs, fungi, and (small) animals that live with and of each other. Whether pine forest or beechwood forest: not only are the trees themselves different, but so is the undergrowth, the leaf litter, and the soil. In each habitat, there is a special community of species, each specifically adapted to the environment and its co-inhabitants. Such a community may seem harmonious on the surface, but is strongly characterized by competition and cooperation. Whoever can best utilize light, water and nutrients, and has cooperative partners who supply them with substances, prevails. Less efficient species have to settle for unattractive niches or are displaced.

As an example of cooperation, the well-known porcini mushroom, which lives in symbiosis with trees, is suitable. Its hyphae encase the fine roots of the partner plants and supply them with water and minerals; in return, it gets sugar delivered from its host. If the cooperation works well, the mushroom can push its delicious fruiting bodies out of the ground in autumn to spread its spores. Also, gut bacteria establish such cooperative relationships by living of metabolic products of other species, offering them advantages in return.

Just as the community of species in forests varies according to environmental conditions, different communities of bacteria also form in humans. Attempts have been made to define different types of such communities as "enterotypes" (Amurugam et al. 2011); however, this view has not prevailed. The conditions on the skin, the mucous membranes or in the gut determine which species can thrive in these biotopes at all. In fact, most body regions are quite inhospitable: On the skin, dryness, high salt content and an acidic environment make survival difficult, the stomach is a pure acid bath, and in the gut, low oxygen, very active digestive enzymes and peristalsis make the body uninhabitable for many bacteria. In addition, the immune system keeps potential interested parties at bay.

Many of the bacterial species that permanently live on and in us have adapted to these harsh conditions over millions of years. As the evolutionary biologist Andrew Moeller from Cornell University in Ithaca has written to me, about a third of the species of human gut bacteria still come from great apes, from which Homo sapiens has evolved. They have opted for a coexistence with humans, and it is likely that this calculation only worked out because the host also benefits from the coexistence.

How the network of bacteria in the human inner ecosystem interacts is still largely unclear. The microbiome of the colon has been most intensively studied, as it is suspected that the causes of many inflammatory and metabolic diseases, as well as digestive disorders, originate here. In addition, stool samples easily reveal information about the inhabitants and, finally, the colon bacteria also make up 99% of the body's bacterial mass. For the species spectrum in the gut, diet plays a crucial role, while genetic influences on the ecosystem are less strong (Goodrich et al. 2014; Gilbert et al. 2018). Thus, identical twins do not always have an identical bacterial flora, as one would expect if their composition were mainly determined by the hosts' genes.

The bacteria optimally adapted to these conditions have the best chances of establishing themselves well and dominating the scene, while other species are less prominent. However, the number of individuals does not always play the biggest role, as bacteria that occur in relatively small numbers often have a key function. These species are referred to as "keystone species". Just like the trees in the forest compete for light, water and good soil, so do the bacteria in the gut compete for nutrients and good conditions. To do this, each elbows its way to secure a good spot with plenty of food. If you manage, as a commensal bacterium, to eliminate the competitors and settle near a nutrient source, you have good chances to thrive. Therefore, many bacteria make life difficult for their foreign neighbors with toxic metabolic products or antibacterial substances, but they also gang up with their clone mates by forming dense colonies, which are referred to as biofilms. However, as a bacterium, you can also team up with other species to better withstand competition.

Unlike a forest, the microbiome does not have a stable environment, but must constantly adapt to changing conditions (different food, diseases, medications, immune response, etc.). This is only achieved by the bacteria constantly receiving stimuli from the host and reacting to them. Optimally adapted inhabitants not only receive signals, but also send out their own to influence the host.

Of Networks, Division of Labor, and Dependencies

The interrelationships between bacterial species establish a complex quasi-social structure in the intestine, with food chains, division of labor, and dependencies. For example, certain bacteria sit directly on the surface of starch granules in the intestinal lumen and gain energy by splitting large starch molecules into fragments, which then dissolve in the fluid of the food pulp. These smaller molecules are further broken down by other bacteria for energy production. This process produces, for example, lactic acid, which is further broken down by other bacteria into short-chain fatty acids, which are utilized by intestinal cells and calm the immune system.

Many bacteria live of the waste products of the species above them in the food chain or exchange substances with partners, similar to how trees cooperate with fungal networks in the soil. There are pronounced dependencies: For example, Faecalibacterium prausnitzii, one of the most common intestinal bacteria, cannot settle by itself in the intestines of mice, but needs the company of other bacteria, preferably bifidobacteria, which produce acetic acid as a waste product. If there are enough bifidobacteria in the environment, Faecalibacterium prausnitzii produces a lot of butyric acid. This substance, in turn, supports the development of regulatory T cells ("Tregs"), which dampen inflammatory responses (Miquel et al. 2014).

Once the right partners have been found in such a network, they form a balance over time through a combination of competition and cooperation, which is not static, but rather changes constantly and dynamically depending on external influences. Of course, such communities always include species that benefit from the services of other species without supporting the network itself. However, it is important that the overall system works.

Bacteria of an ecosystem are also connected through the exchange of genes. In this process, DNA fragments are transferred from one microorganism to another by various mechanisms. If the recipient bacterium benefits from the acquired genes, it can reproduce more effectively. In this way, advantageous characteristics can spread quickly, and it can be observed how the intestinal bacteria of a person optimally adapt to their environment over a few years (Zhao et al. 2019).

For example, in Japan, intestinal bacteria have taken over certain genes from marine bacteria that live in the ocean from algae fibers (Hehemann et al. 2010). Probably, the algae fiber specialists had reached the intestines of humans through sushi or similar foods and their genes were taken over by the resident intestinal bacteria. With this new characteristic, the commensal bacteria could now break down algae fibers and gain energy from them. Since algae are a major part of the daily diet in Japan, the intestinal bacteria upgraded with foreign DNA had an advantage over their competitors and were able to prevail. Therefore, the microbiome of many Japanese people can metabolize carbohydrates from algae that would pass through the intestines of Europeans undigested.

The stability of our inner ecosystem depends largely on the number of bacterial species. If many species are represented in the intestine, and if one species fails, other bacteria can step in. However, if an important species fails in a thinned, species-poor microbiome, the division of labor in the ecosystem can suffer. Other species then no longer receive their important basic substances and also dwindle. Thus, certain, otherwise rather rare bacteria can gain ground, and overweight and digestive and metabolic disorders or inflammations can occur.

Such a "dysbiosis" is observed in inflammatory diseases (Thorburn et al. 2014), but also in overweight, obesity and other diseases of civilization.

However, it is unclear whether and to what extent the disturbed microbiomes are cause or consequence of these diseases. Definitive evidence is still pending, but there is much to suggest a causal relationship (Blaser 2017). The strongest argument is the fact that the microbiome of people living close to nature, who hardly suffer from inflammatory diseases, contains about 60% more bacterial species than is found in people in industrialized countries (Yatsunenko et al. 2012).

Bacteria Everywhere, from Head to Toe

The different areas of the body are specific biotopes, which are used by very different inhabitants. Whether skin, mucous membranes, intestine or internal organs: nutrients, oxygen concentration, salt content or immune responses differ so much that we can say that specialists sit everywhere on and in us, specialists who are adapted to the respective specific conditions and form complex communities with other species.

One of the less attractive habitats for bacteria is the skin. Its surface is not particularly tempting for microorganisms, as it offers relatively few nutrients, is dry in most places and sometimes is salty from sweat. Therefore, only a few bacteria and fungi have settled in this approximately two square meter biotope. These specialists are most likely to liveat the boundaries between cells of the skin surface. Per square centimeter, which is about the area covered by a penny, there are about 100,000 bacteria. About 20 species of known bacteria are commonly found on the skin, including, most commonly, Staphylococcus epidermides and Propionibacterium acnes.

If the skin flora is disturbed, for example, if the skin does not seal tightly due to genetic defects, inflammations or infections, these bacteria can get out of hand. Staphylococci can then penetrate deeper layers of skin and cause inflammation. Propionibacteria are particularly known to multiply in hair follicles filled with fats and waxy substances as a result of hormonal changes during puberty, and can cause acne. Through skin contact, bacteria are easily exchanged between people, so the composition of the skin flora can change very quickly. Whether it results from shaking hands or cuddling, forensic scientists could find this out by comparing the microbiomes of two people.

The bacterial flora of the urogenital tract has been well studied because of its importance for fertility and reproduction, especially in women. In young girls, the vaginal flora consists of a changing mixture of skin and intestinal flora. After the first menstruation, however, almost all women mainly harbor different types of lactobacilli. During pregnancy, the ratio of species changes and the density of the bacterial population increases. This is interpreted as preparation for the colonization of the child during birth.

The lactobacilli live on carbohydrates and sugars, which they convert into lactic acid. The lactic acid results in a relatively acidic pH value of the vagina, which inhibits the growth of pathogenic bacteria. In addition, lactobacilli attack other bacteria using antibacterial molecules and the aggressive chemical hydrogen peroxide. The fact that the surface of the mucous membrane is occupied by such defensive bacteria prevents pathogens from settling.

The bacterial flora of the penis offers far fewer starting points for investigations: It consists of a mixture of different species. Circumcision of the foreskin drastically reduces this diversity.

The respiratory tract has its own microbiome. The upper respiratory tract, i.e., the nose and throat, are lined with an epithelium, that is a tightly sealing cell layer interspersed with mucus cells. These areas are densely populated with commensal bacteria that have an important function: They defend their biotope against invaders, so that bacteria inhaled with the air cannot take hold. A dense colonization is therefore a sign of healthy conditions. Respiratory diseases often go hand in hand with a decline in the healthy bacterial flora. Biological warfare also prevails here: A Tübingen working group has isolated a potent antibiotic from the bacterium Staphylococcus lugdunensis of the nasal cavity, with which the bacterium apparently kills unwanted invaders, and thus keeps competition at bay (Zipperer et al. 2016).

In contrast, the lower respiratory tract, i.e., the trachea and lungs, are relatively poor in bacteria. In healthy individuals, the composition of the bacterial flora of the lower respiratory tract pretty much matches that of the upper respiratory tract, but the total number is lower. Therefore, the inhabitants of the lung are mainly bacteria that have been introduced with the air stream. Apparently, they survive there for a while, but cannot reproduce well and build up dense populations (Man et al. 2017). In diseases with increased mucus production, such as cystic fibrosis or chronic obstructive pulmonary disease (COPD), certain bacteria introduced from the environment appear more frequently.

From the Mouth to the Stomach

As the entrance gate for the digestive tract, the oral cavity is easily accessible to bacteria from the environment, and is therefore very rich in species. Like in the nose, the bacterial flora of the mouth has its biotope firmly in hand and defends it against invaders, so that pathogens have little chance of settling. On one square centimeter of tongue surface, there are about a billion bacteria. One milliliter of saliva, on the other hand, contains a million bacteria. With an average of one liter of saliva that one swallows daily, that's a billion bacteria per day! It has also been calculated that 80 million bacteria are exchanged during a French kiss. Obviously, the exchange of bacteria between humans is very important, otherwise, nature would not have programmed kissing so firmly into our behavior.

Major disturbances can occur when certain commensal bacteria are strongly favored. The prime example for this is caries: By consuming sweets and sugary drinks you fatten up the otherwise rather rare Streptococcus mutans bacteria, which can then assert themselves against other species. They are helped by their ability to communicate with each other and to secrete scaffold substances in which they live in dense colonies. These biofilms are referred to as "plaque" by the dentist. The bacteria sitting in the plaque produce lactic acid, and thus attack the surface of the teeth. This creates holes in the enamel, which can extend through the softer dentin layer into the tooth cavity. The best way to fight this is complete abstinence from sugar, whereby Streptococcus mutans would be at a disadvantage compared to the harmless bacteria.

In the esophagus and stomach, the bacterial flora is less dense and species-rich than in the oral cavity. Because of stomach acid and many antimicrobial substances, the stomach was once considered uninhabited, and it was a surprise to science that bacteria live here nonetheless. However, only one species, the corkscrew-shaped and flagellated bacterium Helicobacter pylori, has conquered this habitat for itself and uses it permanently. The other bacteria found there seem to be rather random short-term guests.

Helicobacter lives in close connection with the cell layer that lines the stomach. The bacterium buffers the stomach acid by producing ammonia with an enzyme, which raises the pH value in the immediate vicinity. In a courageous self-experiment, Barry Marshall was able to prove, in 1984, that this bacterium can cause stomach ulcers: He drank a test tube with a culture of the bacteria and promptly developed a severe gastric mucosal inflammation, which he then cured with antibiotics. Thus, stomach ulcers, which were previously thought to be stress-related, had a bacterial cause! For this finding, he received the Nobel Prize for Medicine in 2005, together with the discoverer of the bacterium, Robin Warren.

Helicobacter pylori can be detected in almost half of all people on this globe, all of whom have a more or less severe gastric mucosal inflammation. Real stomach ulcers develop in about 10–20% of those affected by Helicobacter. Since the infection can lead to stomach cancer, the WHO has classified Helicobacter pylori as carcinogenic. The potential health risk is so great that, in some countries, such as Japan, the eradication of Helicobacter has been planned out. Despite this danger, some scientists, led by the well-known microbiologist Martin Blaser from Rutgers University (New Jersey, USA), attribute an important function to the bacterium in adjusting the immune system. People who are infected with Helicobacter have a lower risk of allergies and asthma—a typical example of a positive side effect, even of pathogens.

The Microbiome of the Gut in Its Habitat

The PubMed database is an indispensable tool for researchers in the biomedical field. Established by the National Library of Congress of the USA in 1970, it provides access to the summaries of 29 million scientific articles published by nearly 5000 journals worldwide. Entered into a search engine, keywords or author names provide information on any conceivable topic at the click of a mouse. If you enter the combination "microbiome" and "gut", the system virtually inundates you with information, listing 40,661 articles. Of these, no fewer than 10,098 articles were published in 2021 (as of March 12, 2022), while, in 2011, there were less than 2%, namely, 144 articles. What could better reflect the immense importance that microbiome research has gained in the last 10 years than this increase in information? There is a veritable explosion of publications, and yet we are only at the beginning of understanding the microbiome. Not surprisingly, the microbiome of the gut takes the most important place, as 99% of the commensal bacteria of humans are gathered there.

Our digestive organ is almost 7 m long in the average adult, with about 5 m for the small intestine and 1.5 m for the large intestine, plus the rectum with almost 20 cm. Between the small and large intestine lies the small appendix of the cecum, which is considered a retreat for bacteria from which they can recolonize the intestine after severe diarrhea or antibiotic treatment.

We tend to count the intestine as part of our inner life, but, on closer inspection, at least its cavity, known as the "lumen", belongs to the outside world. After all, there is a continuous, open connection from the mouth and throat through the stomach and intestine to the anus. Actually, the gastrointestinal tract is a muscular tube that runs like a pipe lengthwise through the body. The food we transport into the acid bath of the stomach by mouth is then directed into the intestine. The small intestine works quickly and hands over its cargo to the large intestine after about 4 h, where the exploitable residues are broken down and metabolized by the gut flora in about a day and a half.

From a bacterial perspective, the intestine is an extreme habitat, which can compete, in terms of hostility to life, with hot springs and glaciers. For example, the atmosphere in the intestinal lumen is practically free of oxygen; fresh air would be deadly for most of our bacterial inhabitants. However, there are also some bacteria that consume the absorbed residual oxygen or use oxygen that diffuses from the blood vessels. Many organisms fail to adapt to harsh conditions such as lack of oxygen, aggressive enzymes, and peristalsis. Thus, 90% of the species of our intestinal bacteria belong to only four of a total of 55 known bacterial major groups (phyla), the already mentioned Firmicutes, Bacteriodetes, Actinobacteria, and Proteobacteria (see the section "A bit of Bacteriology" in Chap. 4). In water or soil, the species diversity is therefore much higher than in the intestine! However, those bacteria that have managed to adapt to the adverse conditions in our interior occur in enormous quantities.

In the small intestine, the colonization density is relatively low, at 10,000 to ten million per milliliter, as it represents a rather bacteria-hostile environment. The conditions in the upper small intestine are particularly harsh, resulting in the lowest density. There, proteins and carbohydrates are digested by aggressive enzymes and bile juice splits fats. The produced nutrients are absorbed by the epithelium and passed on to the blood. To keep bacteria at a distance, the cells of the small intestine in particular constantly produce anti-bacterial substances. Understandably, because the small intestine has little interest in sharing the nutrients just extracted from the food pulp with bacteria.

The situation is quite different in the large intestine. There, the density of bacteria increases to 100 million to 100 billion per milliliter. In a teaspoon of intestinal content, there can therefore be far more bacteria than people on the globe!

In our ingeniously constructed bioreactor, billions of hungry, commensal bacteria pounce on the residues that the human enzymes in the small intestine could not crack and break them down through "fermentation", i.e., enzymatic cleavage under oxygen exclusion. For this, the bacteria are warmed by their human host, regularly supplied with rather liquid food pulp, and given time to work. The human large intestine thus has a function similar to the rumen of ruminants, the difference being that, in the latter, two-thirds of the intestinal tract serve for fermentation, while in humans, it is only about 20%. This reactor exists for a good reason: It provides about 10% of our calories. This may not sound like much, but surely this contribution from our inhabitants was often crucial for surviving dry spells along the path mankind took into the twenty-first century.

Our fermenter is much more than a kind of waste incinerator, in which energy is obtained from residues, because many molecules are also produced there that influence the metabolism, immune system, and nervous system of humans. In the flow-through fermentation chamber, the intestinal bacteria mainly break down complex carbohydrates of plant origin, i.e., certain forms of starch and plant fibers. However, some bacterial species also utilize the carbohydrate-rich intestinal mucus, especially when their plant food becomes scarce. However, even the most diligent intestinal bacteria fail to break down certain plant fibers and other substances. What they leave behind is excreted, along with a bacterial content of about 50%, as feces. Good for research, which thus has plenty of material!

The Intestinal Barrier: More Than an Elastic Wall

Upon closer inspection, the intestine is a marvel! On the one hand, the delicate tube reliably encloses all food components, while, on the other hand, it deliberately channels water and dissolved substances into the body. Solid particles have no access in healthy humans, no matter how small they are. The intestinal wall, a complexly structured mucous membrane underlaid with muscles, protects us from this. Together with chemical and physical components, it forms a tight, but selectively permeable seal against the intestinal lumen, the "intestinal barrier". An inner ring and an outer longitudinal muscle layer enable the churning and squeezing movements of peristalsis, which transport the food pulp through the digestive tract in just under 2 days. The surface of the mucous membrane is so greatly enlarged by tiny, finger-like protrusions, the villi, that it has a total area of about 32 square meters (Helander and Fändricks 2014). Between the intestinal villi are deep indentations, the crypts. At the base of the crypts lie very dividing active stem cells, which provide for a constant renewal of the intestinal epithelium (Fig. 4.3).

The mucous membrane itself consists of delicate and well-blooded connective tissue layers, which are overlaid by a thin layer of cells, the intestinal epithelium. This thin film of cells renews itself completely every 3–4 days and migrates from the crypts to the tips of the villi. At their contact zones, the cells are tightly connected by band-like proteins, almost glued together. This results in a tight seal. Scattered among the actual epithelial cells are goblet cells which secrete viscous mucus. Together with the underlying muscle layers and supporting tissues, the intestinal mucosa and mucus form an elastic cellular wall, which is covered by a layer of mucus.

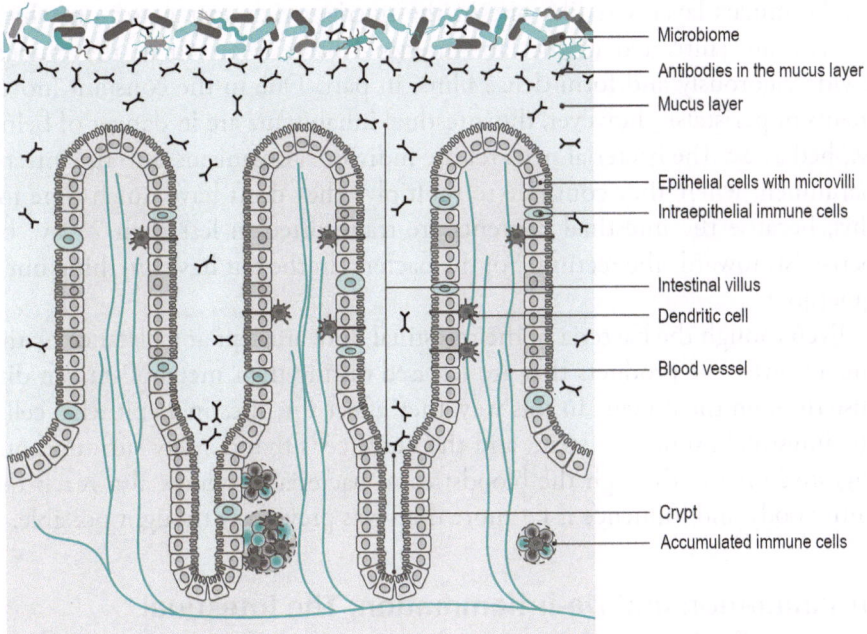

Fig. 4.3 Intestinal villi with overlying mucus layer and intestinal bacteria. The surface of the constantly replenished mucus is grazed by bacteria. Immune cells are located in the intestinal epithelium and below. Details in the text. (Source: Sommer and Bäckhed 2013. © Scorpio Verlag in Europa Verlage GmbH, München. Reproduced with permission)

This mucus, which covers the epithelium as a thin film of about 1/4 millimeter, is an essential element of the intestinal barrier. The mucus consists of proteins with a high proportion of carbohydrates. The huge, long-chain molecules bind water very well. They form a permeable, fluid-filled meshwork, which acts as a sliding layer, allowing the intestinal contents to slide well. In the large intestine, the thin film consists of an upper, quite permeable layer and a lower, very dense layer. Some of the mucus proteins are anchored in the cells of the intestinal epithelium and can receive signals from outside and pass them on to the intestinal cells. The mucus molecules are not attacked by human digestive enzymes, but are an attractive food for some bacteria. Thus, the mucus layer is constantly grazed by intestinal bacteria from the outside and replenished from below by the goblet cells. Antibacterial molecules, supplied by epithelial cells, keep bacteria at a distance. Therefore, most bacteria stay on the surface and penetrate only slightly into the mucus. An intact intestinal barrier, which fulfills its functions despite constant remodeling, is the be-all and end-all for a healthy body.

The mucus layer acts like one of the nutrient-rich agar plates on which bacteria are cultivated in the lab. Intestinal bacteria attach to the mucus, divide vigorously and form dense films, in part. Due to the constant movements of peristalsis, however, the intestinal inhabitants are in danger of being washed away. The bacterial mats release individual organisms into the intestinal lumen, where they continue to multiply. They don't have much time for this, because the intestinal contents are transported in less than 2 days by peristalsis towards the rectum. So, the bacteria in the gut have anything but a quiet job!

Even though the bacteria of the intestinal flora are kept at a distance by the mucus layer, the products that are released during their metabolism can diffuse through the mucus. In this way, they affect the intestinal epithelial cells, the intestinal immune system, and the nerve cells that densely surround our digestive organ. Through the bloodstream, bacterial products also reach the entire body and influence it far more than was previously thought possible.

Inflammation and De-inflammation: The Intestinal Immune System

If you asked students of biology or medicine a few years ago about immunologically important organs, they always mentioned the spleen, bone marrow, or lymph nodes, but never the intestine. A gross misjudgment, because about 70% of all immune cells in the entire body are located in the immediate vicinity of the intestine or directly in the intestinal epithelium! This is no coincidence, as the immune system has essential tasks to perform there: on the one hand, the defense against dangerous pathogens and tumors, against which the immune system proceeds with inflammatory responses, must be carried out. On the other hand, reactions against food components, peaceful commensals, or harmless substances must be avoided and already initiated inflammations must be suppressed. In other words, a de-inflammation must take place.

The fact that this simultaneous control of two opposing processes—fueling and extinguishing inflammation—usually works well is owed largely to our intestinal bacteria. They educate and train the immune system from the first hour of life (see also the excursion "Immune System" in Chap. 8).

The fact that the immune system usually does not attack harmless intestinal inhabitants and food components has been known since the beginning of the twentieth century, but the mechanisms leading to this "immune tolerance" are still not fully understood. It has long been known that you can virtually silence the immune response of mice against any protein by feeding it to the animals. If you inject such pre-treated animals with the protein under the skin, there is hardly any reaction, while the same substance triggers a violent inflammation in control animals. This effect is known as "oral tolerance" (Weiner et al. 2011). Apparently, the recognition of harmless molecules in the intestine by the immune system leads to reactions that prevent inflammation from the outset. The inflammation brake triggered in the intestine affects the entire body, as immune cells are very migratory and take their inhibitory message with them. This immune tolerance is as important for our survival as the defense against pathogens, because we are constantly confronted with myriads of different harmless substances through the skin, the mucous membranes, and the intestine. All these substances, and even the body's own molecules, could trigger inflammation if it weren't for the inhibitory mechanisms.

The cells of the intestinal immune system responsible for promoting or inhibiting inflammation are either organized in groups or reside individually in the tissue under the intestinal epithelium and in the epithelium itself, while many are also gathered in lymph nodes. They constantly monitor the intestinal contents. An important role is played by a special type of phagocyte, the dendritic cells: They sit directly beneath the intestinal epithelium, extend their processes like the tentacles of an octopus through gaps between the cells and take samples from the intestinal lumen. They digest the ingested substances and present protein fragments of them to the most important control cells of the immune system, the T cells (Fig. 4.4). This presentation programs the T cells and enables them to release their immune messenger substances, the "cytokines", either fueling or inhibiting inflammation.

Immune tolerance is achieved by the immune system in the healthy gut by reacting to molecules from food and components of the gut flora with inhibitory responses, rather than triggering inflammation. The mechanisms differ in the individual sections of the gut. In the small intestine, the inhibitory effect is predominantly created as a result of the contact with foreign substances stimulating T cells so strongly that they activate a suicide program and disintegrate into their components (Visekruna et al. 2019; Rodriguez-Sillke et al. 2021). Thus, immune responses are prevented from the outset without significant involvement of the microbiome.

The inhibition of inflammatory responses in the colon (Fig. 4.4) occurs quite differently. When dendritic cells are under the influence of certain bacterial metabolic products, the short-chain fatty acids, during the presentation of protein fragments, they program T cells towards immune tolerance. These small molecules are produced by certain bacteria during the breakdown of complex carbohydrates (see the following section "Dietary Fibers"). Under their influence, the dendritic cells cause the previously mentioned regulatory

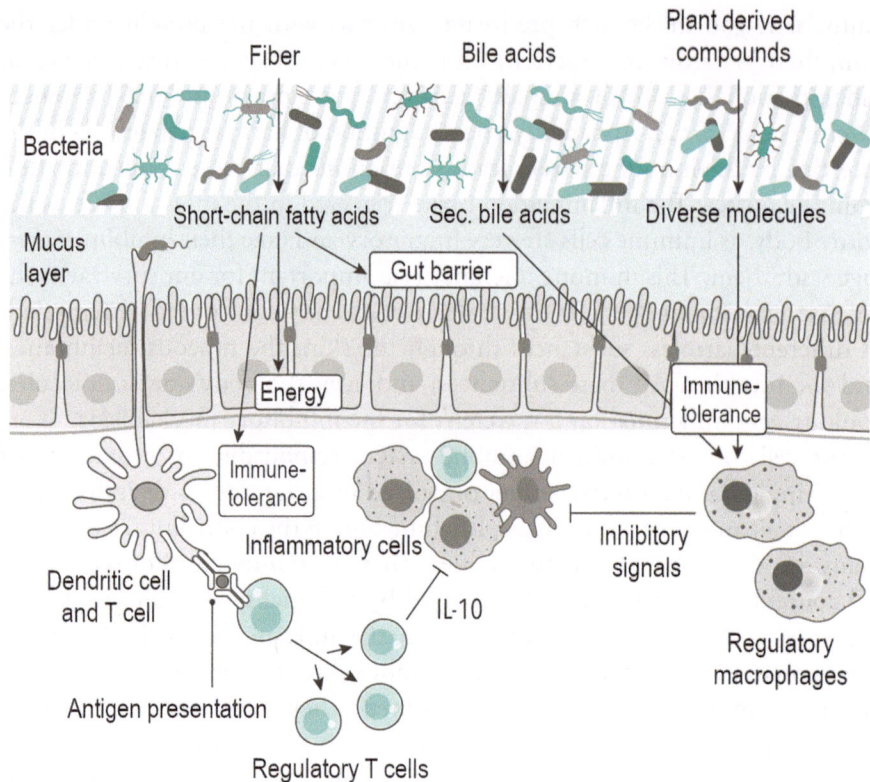

Fig. 4.4 Development of immune tolerance through the influence of bacterial metabolites. Gut bacteria produce short-chain fatty acids by breaking down complex carbohydrates, which influence dendritic cells. During antigen presentation, these program T cells into regulatory T cells (Tregs), whose offspring downregulate the inflammatory process with cytokines such as IL-10. Secondary bile acids and metabolites of plant constituents also have anti-inflammatory effects. (© Scorpio Verlag in Europa Verlage GmbH, München. Reproduced with permission)

T cells or "Tregs" to develop. These regulators multiply strongly and inhibit inflammatory reactions throughout the body by releasing anti-inflammatory cytokines (Kim et al. 2016). As the "peacekeeping force of the immune system", they calm other immune cells, and thus act as an inflammation brake.

Repeated contact with substances from food or with bacterial components strengthens—similarly to a vaccination—the inhibitory responses of the Tregs, and thus consolidates immune tolerance (Rosenblum et al. 2015). If the production of short-chain fatty acids by gut bacteria is lacking, the effect of the inflammation brake decreases. In addition, other metabolic products of bacteria (Wang et al. 2019) and components of food, such as omega-3 fatty acids, suppress inflammatory responses in the gut in various ways. The impact of food on immune responses is also addressed in Chap. 6 "Food" and in the excursion "Macro and Micronutrients" in Chap. 8.

Our Gut Brain

Once a modern long-haul jet has taken off and the pilot has switched to automatic flight control, they may not have to intervene in the control for hours. The computer system constantly receives information from sensors and instruct the autopilot on position, air currents, temperature, fuel consumption, and other details. These signals are integrated and result in instructions to adjust the elevators, extend the landing flaps, or the pilot is informed about the fuel tank level. As long as the automatic control is engaged, the pilots essentially only have to monitor the system and intervene in critical situations.

Similarly, the processes of digestion are controlled by an autonomous system consisting of about 200 million nerve cells that surround the intestine as a dense network. It is connected to the brain by thick nerve strands that transmit information in both directions. The "enteric nervous system" consists of only one thousandth of the number of cells that our brain has, but our "gut brain" nevertheless performs astonishing feats. After all, its number of cells corresponds to that of a cat's brain.

Our" second brain" constantly collects immense amounts of information from the intestine and the entire body, integrates them, and initiates corresponding activities as needed. These pieces of information naturally include signals originating from the microbiome in the intestine. Thus, the gut flora continuously communicates with the nervous system and can influence control processes in this way. When we have a" gut feeling", that is, make an intuitive decision without engaging the mind, it could well be that the bacteria in the intestine are exerting their influence.

However, the prosaic tasks of the enteric nervous system are usually at the forefront: Over the course of an 80-year life, the intestine processes more than 30 tons of food and 50,000 liters of liquid. The enteric nervous system controls this enormous throughput. Alone the task to transport these masses is immense: All this material must be pumped from the stomach towards the anus by the kneading movements of peristalsis. Whether a meal is fatty and the gallbladder must secrete fluid, whether the food pulp in the intestine needs to be transported further or the blood flow needs to be increased: The gut brain regulates these processes. The control center analyzes nutrient composition and salt content, controls the balances of messenger substances, and communicates with the immune system. This data processing, which runs continuously day and night, is fully automatic.

Under normal conditions, different programs of the gut brain are active, depending on whether and what food was consumed, whether one is resting or active, asleep or awake. Most of the information accessed by the enteric nervous system comes from a multitude of sensors on the intestinal surface that constantly analyze the filling state of the intestine and the taste, consistency, fat content, and other properties of the intestinal contents, and determine which food is currently being processed. For example, when the fat content is high, the secretion of bile fluid is stimulated and the emptying of the stomach and the passage through the intestine are slowed down. However, when the receptors sense glucose, they stimulate the absorption of the sugar into the blood and simultaneously increase the production of insulin by the pancreas, so that the energy supplier is absorbed into cells. In its activities, the enteric nervous system keeps the brain, as the superior control center, informed and, for example, tells it when food is needed. Thus, the brain can get its owner moving by releasing hunger hormones that stimulate it to get food. Conversely, a hormonally controlled feeling of satiety from the stomach tells the brain that it would be better to skip a second serving of dessert.

However, the brain retains supremacy and, if necessary, instructs the enteric nervous system to interrupt its routine. A very impressive example was described to me by a colleague: On a trip to the Galapagos Islands, he contracted persistent, severe diarrhea for days from a delicious avocado salad that was apparently contaminated with salmonella. This "Montezuma's revenge" was a reaction of the body meant to get rid of the bacteria. The brain remembered the connection between avocado and danger and, from then on, reliably instructed the enteric nervous system to switch to diarrhea at the sight of avocados. Even 30 years later, my colleague avoids the fruit and vegetable sections of supermarkets to avoid this danger! In a similar way, the brain interrupts the digestion programs during fear and flight reactions. Instead, it instructs the enteric nervous system to start up the intestinal motor in order to shed ballast for a possible necessary flight.

Our gut bacteria are connected, in many ways, to this on-board computer, and also to the brain. As gastroenterologist Emeran Mayer vividly describes in his book "The Second Brain" (2016), bacteria and humans share a common language. Essentially—according to Mayer—many of the body's messenger substances are ancient inventions of bacteria, which we have retained over the course of evolution because they were successful. It is precisely these conserved substances that our commensal bacteria use to play on the keyboard of the enteric nervous system, the brain, and the immune system. Often, they play indirectly, influencing the immune system with their products, which, in turn, affects the gut brain. Such signals are then passed on to the brain via the vagus nerve, which then initiates fever and sleep. In inflammatory diseases, this reaction causes the constant fatigue from which many patients suffer (Browning et al. 2017).

In Constant Change

Our Bacterial Community: The Legacy of Many Generations

Each person has their own, individual gut flora, which is typical for them, so that the patterns of species and of their quantities are different from that of their neighbors. Therefore, the comparison with a personal fingerprint is not entirely far-fetched. Forensic scientists are also flirting with the possibility of identifying perpetrators based on the composition of bacterial species at a crime scene. Within a family living together, and even within a rental house, more similarities will be found than with strangers, yet the bacterial communities of family members also differ from each other. Even identical twins can have a different microbiome, as genetic influences are not predominant. The composition of the gut flora is essentially shaped in the first 3 years of life. After that, humans and bacterial communities have adapted to each other and the balance remains largely stable unless living conditions change substantially.

A newborn human receives its bacterial starter kit in the form of lactobacilli from the mother's birth canal mucous membranes, but also from her skin and gut microbiome (Ferretti et al. 2018). The baby is literally inoculated with the mother's bacteria. The first settlers are lactobacilli from the maternal vaginal flora, which enter the newborn's mouth during the birth process. Since the intestines are also pressed during labor, it is quite normal for a newborn to also become acquainted with the mother's gut bacteria.

The first bacteria help determine who can subsequently settle in the gut. The dense population of lactobacilli produces so much lactic acid that other species can hardly gain a foothold. The next settlers are bifidobacteria, which are not deterred by the acidic environment and settle in the infant's gut. Other bacteria that settle in the child's digestive tract come from breast milk and the microbiome of other people and contribute over time to the development of a healthy, diverse community of species. By the third year of life, a complex microbiome has developed, as is typical for adults.

The importance of the type of first colonization of a newborn is shown by studies on children born through cesarean section. A Danish study followed the medical histories of 2 million children and found that cesarean section children are more likely to suffer from asthma and chronic inflammatory bowel diseases later in life compared to vaginally born children (Sevelsted et al. 2015). This increased disease risk is attributed to the fact that, after a cesarean section, the number of bacterial species in the gut is lower and more potentially pathogenic germs occur than in vaginally born infants. Apparently, the early childhood microbiome shapes the immune system and helps to establish immune tolerance later in life.

Breastfeeding also shows how closely humans and their commensal bacteria are adapted to each other. Nutrition from breast milk promotes many types of bifidobacteria in the first months of life, and these can make up the majority of the microbiome in breastfed children. Here, one can directly speak of a cultivation of the right bacteria: breast milk contains—and this is no coincidence—certain, complex sugar molecules, the "human milk oligosaccharides" = HMO. These molecules are the third most important component of breast milk after lactose and fat. They cannot be used at all by the digestive system of the toddler, but they are feed for bifidobacteria. The bacteria break down the HMOs and, in the process, produce short-chain fatty acids, which provide energy and calm the immune system of the infant and program it for immune tolerance. The mother thus not only feeds her child, but also shapes its emerging microbiome. There are over 200 variants of HMOs, the ratio of which changes during breastfeeding. As a result, the bacterial flora also changes and optimally matches the respective developmental stage of the child.

With breast milk, not only is bacteria feed provided, but gut bacteria are also specifically transferred from the mother to the child. Until recently, it was believed that such bacteria from the area around the nipples would get into the mouth of the infant. However, it has now been demonstrated in mice that lactobacilli from the mother animal's gut reach the young mice's gut via the milk gland (De Andres et al. 2017). Many findings suggest a very similar process in humans (Rodriguez et al. 2021). In a study of Guatemalan mothers, whose milk microbiome was analyzed over the course of 6 months, the spectrum of transferred bacterial species also changed during breastfeeding (Gonzales et al. 2021), another indication of the sophisticated mechanisms that ensure an optimal microbiome for the toddler. Off-the-shelf baby food is usually of less high-quality in comparison, because it does not contain HMOs. Consequently, the gut flora of bottle-fed children contains only about half as many bifidobacteria as that of those fed with breast milk (Rinninella et al. 2019).

Food and environment populate the infant's, and later the toddler's, gut with additional bacteria. In the gut, species that have been ingested with pre-chewed food, drink, or swallowed mucus from their own respiratory tract find conditions that are suitable to varying degrees. Depending on competition from other bacteria, food supply, immune status, and other factors, they can then settle and establish themselves more or less successfully. So, why shouldn't healthy parents suck off their baby's pacifier? They are in close contact with the child anyway and their bacteria are incorporated into its microbiome.

Family members, pets, and the environment are constantly providing commensal bacteria. Consequently, the gut microbiome can reveal whether people live together in a household. Humans also take bacteria from dogs and livestock into their microbiome (Song et al. 2013; Sun et al. 2020). Surely, the pronounced behavior of toddlers to put all reachable objects in their mouths also contributes to populating the gut with a diverse bacterial flora. Toddlers in the crawling stage explore their environment almost entirely with their mouths!

From about the third year of life, a fairly stable gut flora has established itself, lasting into old age if diet and environmental conditions remain similar. Difficulties can arise when the balance among the species is disturbed. This is particularly the case after repeated antibiotic treatments, which swirl in confusion the species composition each time they are administered. Then, certain species of bacteria have to step back or disappear, and others spread. Usually, however, the system will settle back into a stable state after some time. However, species can be lost in the process.

With the loss of bacterial species, the risk for inflammatory diseases increases (Gensollen et al. 2016). In this context, it is alarming that people in affluent societies already have a less diverse gut flora in their normal state. Children of mothers with thinned-out microbiomes "inherit" relatively few bacterial species from the outset. If their gut flora is further depleted by unbalanced nutrition, improper antibiotic treatment, or other factors, the shaping of the immune system, and thus the development of immune tolerance, suffers.

In older age, the average diversity of species in the gut decreases in Western societies. Often, harmful and inflammation-promoting bacteria increase, which could explain the tendency of aging people to inflammation. Immunologists sometimes refer to this process as "inflammaging", or "inflammatory aging". This tendency also depends on the living conditions of the elderly, and particularly on their diet. Especially in nursing homes, where "easily digestible" food that should not strain the gut is often served, the microbiome becomes thinned-out. In traditionally living societies, where the elderly are not so isolated, are more involved in daily activities and have more contact with environmental bacteria, these changes are not so pronounced (Fragiadakis et al. 2019).

Meat or Vegetables: The Influence of Nutrition

A steppe region in Tanzania, right next to the world-famous Serengeti National Park, is home to a people of hunter-gatherers, the Hadza. Now pushed back to a few barren areas, there are still a few hundred people here who have maintained the lifestyle of their ancestors. The small, slender Hadza, who belong to the original African population, live in simple huts made of branches and gather and hunt their food directly in the savannah. Since there are pronounced seasons in East Africa, the food supply changes seasonally. In the rainy season, the food is varied, with berries, fruits, wild vegetables, small animals, and honey. In the dry season, the offer is sparse, but larger game is hunted, and more meat is eaten, as the animals are drawn to the few water holes and can be killed more easily. Starchy root tubers, which the Hadza resort to when other food is scarce, can be found all year round.

These "Last of the First", as a documentary calls the Hadza, have been well studied in terms of ancestry, language, health, and traditions, and are therefore something like a model case of a hunter-gatherer society. In recent years, they have also attracted the attention of nutrition and microbiome researchers, in particular, the couple Justin and Erica Sonnenburg, who lead a very productive working group at Stanford University, one of the American research Eldorados. By studying a natural people, a window into the past opens up, and one can imagine how our ancestors ate, how their microbiome was composed, and how it reacted to changes in the food supply.

The data from the Sonnenburgs show that part of the Hadza's microbiome is in constant flux. When the hunters are successful in the dry season and bring home a lot of game, bacteria that thrive on a meat diet multiply. They grow into dense populations, while the specialists in the utilization of plant fibers do not thrive well and lead a niche existence. Conversely, when vegetarian food flows through the digestive tract for a longer period of time, the bacteria specialized in a meat diet have a hard time and grow slower than competitors who love plant residues. In the gut, the same competitive relationships exist as in other ecosystems: those who adapt best to changing conditions thrive. However, there is a core of species that are "generalists", which can live under all conditions, and are therefore constantly present in the microbiome.

Naturally, it is of great interest to analyze the change of bacterial populations under precisely defined conditions. In an impressive study from the group led by Peter Turnbaugh (David et al. 2014) at Harvard University, the scientists asked six men and four women, who were used to a mixed diet, to eat either purely animal or exclusively plant-based diets for five consecutive days. During this time and a subsequent observation phase of 6 days, the subjects had to continuously provide stool samples. The gut flora responded to this change within 2 days.

The strongest effect was a switch to a purely animal diet: Such an extreme diet is hard on many bacterial species, whose populations then shrink, while a few species benefit from the new situation and spread. Why? A diet that consists only of animal products promotes the production of aggressive bile juices, which break down fats, but can also attack certain bacteria. Therefore, bacteria that are resistant to bile juice and can metabolize proteins benefited from the change. The switch to a purely plant-based diet had less pronounced changes. Just 2 days after the end of the experiment, after the subjects had returned to their usual diet, their gut flora had returned to its original state.

This impressively demonstrated how quickly the human microbiome reacts to changes in diet. But how does this finding correlate with the fact that the gut microbiome of an adult human is relatively stable? One reason is that many bacteria can adapt their programs for food utilization within a limited range to the circumstances. They either have built-in alternative genetic programs that can be activated as needed, or they acquire genes from other bacteria. Thus, they can thrive again after a period of suffering. Overall, however, changes in dietary patterns in affluent societies are not too frequent, as several nutrition experts have confirmed to me. Most well-intentioned people who want to switch to a different diet are usually back to their old preferences after a few months. Could it be that one has an involuntary need to come into a state of equilibrium with one's accustomed microbiome?

Similar to the composition of the diet, medications can also affect the microbiome of the gut. The team led by Peer Bork at the European Molecular Biology Lab (EMBL) in Heidelberg examined the impact of more than 1000 commercially available drugs from human and veterinary medicine on the growth of 40 representative strains of gut bacteria (Maier et al. 2018). 24% of these drugs inhibited the growth of at least one bacterial strain. In particular, tumor-inhibiting substances and, notably, many psychotropic drugs slowed the growth of bacteria. Therefore, it is expected that these medications also cause lasting shifts in the species composition of the gut flora. In fact, for some drugs, there is reason to believe that part of their effect is due to the altered microbiome (Nayak et al. 2021). Like medications, chemicals such as emulsifiers, synthetic sweeteners and other food additives also influence the microbiome, but the effects are rarely known, as shown in Chap. 6 on the topic of food.

Dietary Fiber: Favorite Food of the Gut Flora

In order to grow and reproduce, bacteria break down various substances to derive energy from them. For the human gut flora, carbohydrates are the most important food. For their breakdown, the bacteria have a huge variety of enzymes at their disposal: The gut flora as a whole has thousands of these digestive helpers, while the human intestine itself can only use 17 different enzymes to break down carbohydrates (El Kaoutary et al. 2013). No wonder, then, that, in the small intestine, after the digestion of sugars and simple carbohydrates, fats and proteins, many complex carbohydrates remain. These residues, which are indigestible for the human intestine, are referred to as dietary fiber. These can be coarser components of plants, such as fibers, structural substances or cell walls, but also soluble carbohydrates like pectin or inulin. These dietary fibers are essentially made up of long chains of different sugar molecules, the breakdown of which provides bacteria with energy.

Dietary fiber has long been known to promote digestion by stimulating bowel activity, binding water, and thus giving the stool its consistency. But it has also other important functions: Dietary fiber is a source of short-chain fatty acids. These small molecules, which include acetic acid, propionic acid and butyric acid, are produced by certain types of bacteria during the breakdown of plant substances. They have a strong smell and are volatile. Anyone who has ever smelled rancid butter knows what I'm talking about. On the one hand, butyric acid & Co. are used by intestinal cells or in the liver as a source of energy and, in this way, contribute about 10% of human calories. In the rocky phases of its development, Homo sapiens would probably have been left behind more often without their intestinal bacteria and the calories they provide.

Another function of short-chain fatty acids cannot be overestimated: They are calming pills for the immune system. If the intestinal bacteria release enough short-chain fatty acids, they reprogram—as previously described—the development of T cells. Then, regulatory T cells are formed that inhibit inflammatory processes with their messenger substances.

To ensure an adequate supply of short-chain fatty acids, a balanced diet is important, one that is rich in plant-based dietary fiber. Vegetables, fruits and whole grain products should therefore definitely be an important part of the diet.

If the diet lacks dietary fiber, the bacteria starve and have to resort to the carbohydrate-rich mucus that lines the colon as an emergency ration. This meager food produces fewer short-chain fatty acids, thus providing fewer calming pills for the immune system. In addition, a thin, nibbled mucus layer only imperfectly shields the intestine from pathogens, and thus promotes inflammation. An adequate supply of dietary fiber is therefore a prerequisite for sufficient production of tolerance-promoting short-chain fatty acids. It is best to also ensure a lot of variety in the bacteria's food (see also the excursus "Macronutrients and Micronutrients" in Chap. 8). Then, a diverse, versatile bacterial flora can thrive, as is typical for people in pre-industrial societies.

The Microbiome of Our Ancestors

If you want to know how the microbiomes of our early ancestors were composed, you are essentially dependent on comparisons with microbiomes of people who live under similar conditions today as humans did in earlier millennia. In feces, DNA decomposes very quickly and, so far, no material has been found in Neanderthal sites or Stone Age graves that would be suitable for microbiome analyses. However, in a few cases, bacterial DNA could be isolated: from 1000- to 2000-year-old human feces from extremely dry regions in the southern USA and in Mexico. The microbiomes from these fecal samples resemble those of today's hunters and gatherers (Wibowo et al. 2021).

This is anything but a surprise, as the first modern humans, who emerged about 250,000 years ago, probably lived and fed similarly to the last existing indigenous peoples today. Therefore, studies on the microbiome of such societies living close to nature provide a glimpse into the past. A good example is the microbiomes of Guahibo Indians in Venezuela, who live as hunters and gatherers in the rainforest. In them, the number of bacterial species of the gut microbiome is, on average, 63% higher than in residents of the USA. The species diversity in a comparison group of traditionally living Africans, who mainly fed on corn, was still 33% above the value of the Americans (Yatsunenko et al. 2012). The highest species diversity of the gut microbiome was found in Yanomami Indians from rainforest areas in Venezuela, people had never before been in contact with Western civilization (Clemente et al. 2015) (Fig. 4.5).

The internal species diversity in hunters and gatherers is not surprising, given the very varied diet and constant contact with bacteria from soil, animals, plants, and untreated water. The diversity of food plants alone, with their specific structural and content substances, probably keeps a whole armada of different bacterial species alive. In addition, in the microbiomes of people living close to nature, bacterial species and groups appear that are almost never found in the microbiome of modern city dwellers. These exotics

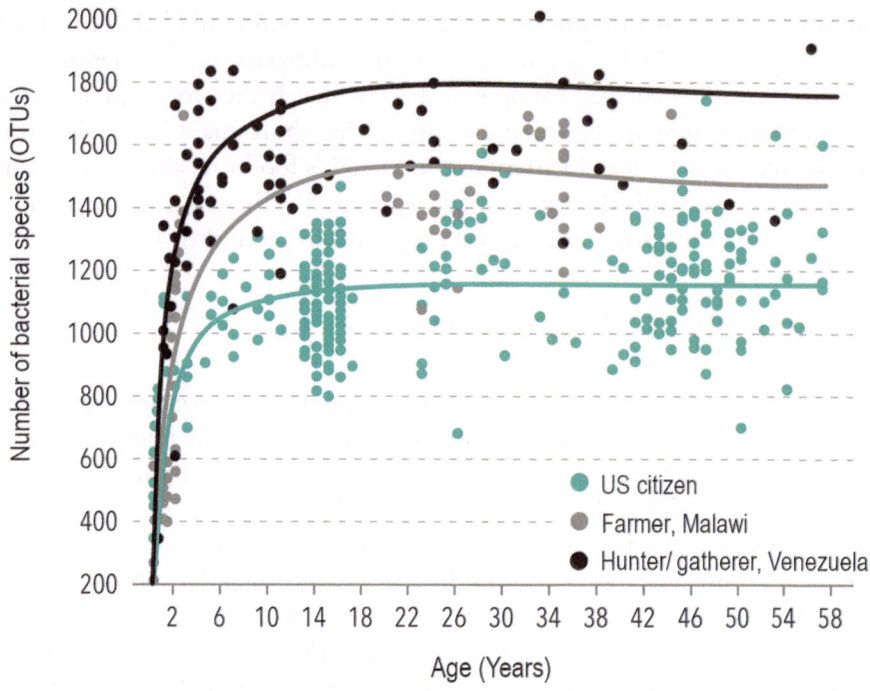

Fig. 4.5 Comparison of the diversity of human microbiomes with different lifestyles. The number of gut bacteria increases in childhood and then reaches a plateau. In the Guahibo Indians (hunters and gatherers, Venezuela), it is 63% higher, and in African farmers (Malawi), 31% higher than in residents of the USA. The lines indicate averages. (Modified after Yatsunenko et al. 2012. © Scorpio Verlag in Europa Verlage GmbH, München. Reproduced with permission)

include species of spirochetes and succinivibrions, which are probably specialists in the breakdown of certain plant fibers (Obregon-Tito et al. 2015). With the increasing change in lifestyle, we have apparently lost more and more of this internal species diversity on the way to the "western lifestyle" and now rely on a gut flora that only masters the standard tasks.

In this context, it is interesting that, in traditionally living societies, with their species-rich microbiomes, diet-related diseases are very rare. The well-known tropical medicine specialist Burkitt described this connection as early as the 1970s in numerous articles (O'Keefe 2019). Just like those in the previously mentioned "Blue Zones", their lifestyle seems to protect people from these ailments. A less opulent diet, lots of exercise and contact with nature mean that, contrary to popular belief, people in traditional societies often reach a high age of 68–78 years (Gurven and Kaplan 2007). Those who have survived early childhood with its infections and the dangerous teenage years can indeed become very old, because obesity and chronic diseases are insignificant as causes of death in such societies (Carrera-Bastos et al. 2011).

Even though the diet and environmental influences that affect the microbiome of humans are very different worldwide, there are about 50 "core species" of bacteria that occur in almost all humans. However, their frequency distribution varies greatly according to dietary and lifestyle habits. Humans apparently maintain a very long-standing collaboration with these gut bacteria, while other bacterial species have only joined us later. We have probably been living with the core species for millions of years. Molecular family trees show that the commensal bacteria of humans have common roots with the gut bacteria of today's primates.

Compared to our ape relatives, humans have the poorest microbiome (Moeller et al. 2017). This loss of species probably began when the genus Homo entered the scene about 2.5 million years ago. When the great apes split into different species about 30 million years ago, their gut bacteria also evolved into different directions. Thus, gorillas, chimpanzees, bonobos (dwarf chimpanzees), and humans each have their own set of standard bacterial pets, which are closely adapted to the respective host species, as evolutionary biologist Andrew Moeller of Cornell University in Ithaca, NY, USA, notes (Moeller et al. 2016). Their transmission mainly occurs through body contact from mother to child. Approximately one third of the microbial species diversity in the human gut is derived from its primate ancestors, according to Moeller. Two thirds are of other origins, having been acquired from the environment or perhaps other animals over the course of evolution.

Against the backdrop of this long coexistence, the sophisticated influence of bacteria on the human body and brain becomes very plausible. If we have been living with certain bacteria for hundreds of thousands of generations, there has been ample time to adjust to each other. An example is the particularly well-studied bacteria of the genus Bacteroides, which break down carbohydrates and proteins. A very close cooperation has developed with them through joint evolution, a fact that can be read from the enzyme equipment of the bacteria.

For example, about two thirds of the carbohydrate-digesting enzymes of the well-studied model organism Bacteroides thetaiotaomicron break down plant starch, but one third is specialized in carbohydrates of the intestinal mucus. Over the course of its millions of years of coexistence with the host, the bacterium has diversified its eating utensils so that it can utilize this diverse diet. When the menu offers plant starch, the specialized enzymes of the generalist work and crack starch molecules. When there is no starch on offer, B. thetaiotaomicron produces alternative enzymes and switches to intestinal mucus as a food source. Then, the bacteria graze the surface of the mucus layer, which the host constantly replenishes. However, the bacterium then tells the intestine to please incorporate an additional special sugar, which it can utilize particularly well, into the carbohydrates of the mucus. The goblet cells then activate an otherwise inactive gene and secrete—as ordered by B. thetaiotaomicron—sugared mucus. But the signals also go in the opposite direction: In response to certain stimuli, B. thetaiotaomicron changes its surface molecules to adapt to the host's immune responses (Porter et al. 2018).

How intensively humans interact with their gut bacteria is also shown by the previously mentioned example of bifidobacteria, which are among the first colonizers of the infant gut and live on carbohydrates specially produced for them in breast milk. Bifido- and Bacteroides bacteria are probably among our oldest and closest cooperation partners. Bacteria of the genus Prevotella, which break down complex carbohydrates from plant fibers, also belong to the core population of the human microbiome, but are strongly pushed back by the Western diet (Tett et al. 2021). Other gut bacteria have arrived later and then settled in. One of these latecomers could be Ruminococcus bromii, which can make up a significant portion of the gut flora not only in humans, but also in cattle (Mukhopadhya et al. 2018).

Stone Age Gut and the Western Diet

About 10,000 years ago, there was a tremendous upheaval in human history following climate changes, the "Neolithic Revolution". In the Neolithic Age, people transitioned from a life as nomadic hunters and gatherers to agriculture and livestock farming—independently of each other in such different regions of the world as the Near East, South China, Central America, and West Africa.

The diet spectrum changed dramatically, as, instead of root tubers, seeds, insects, nuts, wild vegetables, fish, and lean game meat, people now primarily consumed grain products or starchy plant tubers. People became sedentary, which facilitated the domestication of animals such as goats, sheep, and cattle. Agriculture laid the foundation for denser settlements and villages, and cities emerged. In typical agricultural societies, the proportion of animal proteins in the diet decreased compared to the earlier hunter-gatherer cultures, and the food became less varied. The new lifestyle could feed more people, but they were not necessarily better off, as the average body size decreased compared to hunters and gatherers, as skeletal finds from this time prove.

Agriculture and livestock farming not only fundamentally changed the human diet, but also the human microbiome. Overall, the menu of peasant societies became more monotonous and uniform, so fewer bacterial specialists were needed for special tasks. The grinding of grain and cooking of food also reduced those bacterial species that specialize in the breakdown of very resistant plant components. This is reflected in a comparison between microbiomes of currently living hunters and gatherers on the one hand and traditionally living farmers on the other: In societies that mainly practice agriculture and eat a predominantly vegetarian diet, carbohydrate-utilizing bacteria are strongly represented. Typical of this are Prevotella and Xylanibacter, which ferment complex carbohydrates from plants (De Filippo et al. 2010).

But not only has the microbiome changed since the Neolithic, but so has the human digestive system, as genetic analyses show. With the advent of agriculture, grains and other starchy plant products became the main source of energy. Therefore, people in whom mutations of digestive enzymes led to a more efficient digestion of starch now had better chances of surviving and reproducing—the corresponding gene variants consequently increased in the population. Similar adaptations to new dietary habits also occurred in societies where dairy farming played a major role. The original blueprint of the mammal human stipulates that only the intestine of children has an enzyme equipment that allows for the digestion of milk. As an adult, one is actually lactose intolerant, so that consumption of milk leads to bloating and digestive disorders. However, those who could still digest milk and dairy products well beyond childhood and cover their protein needs from this source had a vital advantage. Therefore, in Northern Europe, the frequency of people in whom the milk-digesting enzyme lactase is still produced by adults increased (Walter and Ley 2019).

The dietary change already completed in industrialized countries and currently taking place in the rest of the world represent a second dietary revolution. As a main trait, people shifted from self-sufficiency to industrial nutrition. Hand in hand with the changes in food went the use of antibiotics and drugs, highly developed hygiene and the decline in contact with nature. How quickly the transition to Western living conditions changes the microbiome is shown by a study conducted with Asian immigrants in the USA. Just 9 months after arrival in the USA, the microbiome of the immigrants had changed, with the frequency of Prevotella bacteria, which break down plant fibers, decreasing in favor of Bacteroides. At the same time, the diversity of species decreased and rare bacteria, which are typical for a close-to-nature lifestyle, disappeared. This development intensified with the increasing length of the stay and took place over decades. The microbiome of second-generation immigrants no longer differed significantly from that of native US citizens (Vangay et al. 2018).

As a result of their western lifestyle, as previously mentioned, modern city dwellers have a significantly less diverse microbiome than hunters and gatherers, or people from traditional agricultural societies. Unsurprisingly, the microbiome of modern city dwellers contains many species of bacteria that can efficiently metabolize sugar and other readily available carbohydrates and are resistant to bile, which is secreted in greater amounts during fatty meals. These species thrive on a diet of sweet and fatty, industrially produced foods that satisfy our evolutionarily conditioned hunger for calorie-rich food. Bacteria of the Firmicutes group find particularly good living conditions, as a comparison between African and European microbiomes shows (De Filippo et al. 2010, Fig. 4.6). The fact that some Firmicutes species form resistant spores that can be easily transmitted despite hygiene may have contributed to their flourishing in modern societies.

The degree to which the inner ecosystem of people in industrialized countries has changed is shown by a very interesting study from the research group led by Andrew Moeller: They compared the microbiomes of residents of the

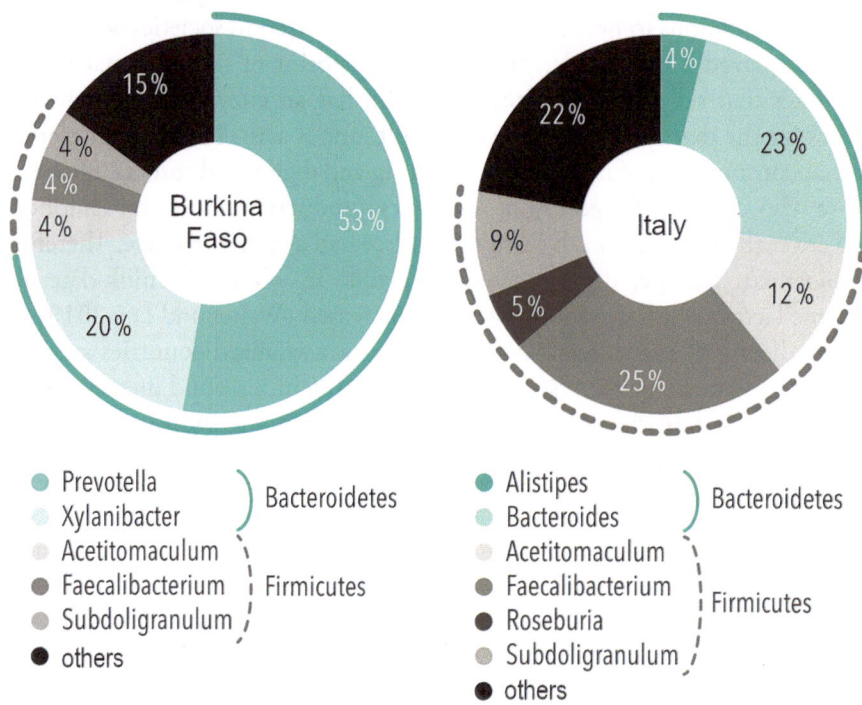

Fig. 4.6 Composition of the gut microbiome of children from Burkina Faso (West Africa) and Italy. In the gut of African children, Bacteroidetes bacteria, which break down plant fibers, dominate, while in the gut of Italian children, Firmicutes bacteria, typical for the western lifestyle, predominate. (Modified after De Filippo et al. 2010. © Scorpio Verlag in Europa Verlage GmbH, München. Reproduced with permission)

USA, people living close to nature in Venezuela and Malawi, and great apes (bonobos, chimpanzees, gorillas). They quantified the evolutionary distance in a distance matrix. A kind of triangular relationship emerged, with very clear differences: The microbiomes of great apes and US residents were very far apart, while the gut flora of people living close to nature was in the middle between the two extremes (Fig. 4.7). Accordingly, the difference between the gut flora of people living close to nature and US residents was similar to that between great apes and people living close to nature. The data suggest that the transition from a person living close to nature to a city dweller with a western lifestyle has changed the microbiome as much as the transition from a great ape to a person living close to nature has (Moeller et al. 2014).

The remarkable thing about this triangular image of microbiomes is the time span that lies between the point clouds. While the development from the ape microbiome to that of humans took about 5 million years, the change from the microbiome of the person living close to nature to the microbiome of the modern city dweller occurred comparatively instantaneously, in only about 60 years. With the introduction of industrially produced food, fast food, sugary drinks, and medications, humans have massively changed the basis of life of their microbiome. As a result, new bacteria have spread that do

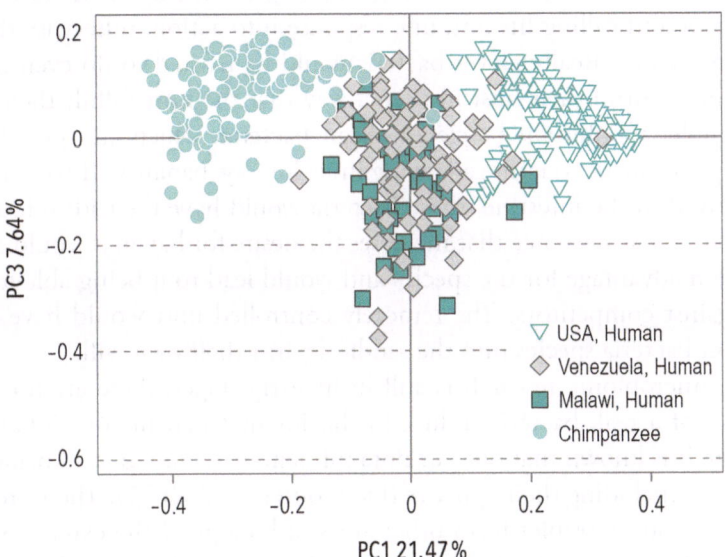

Fig. 4.7 Comparison of microbiomes through a distance matrix. The microbiomes of chimpanzees (left), people living close to nature in South America and Africa (center), and US citizens with a western lifestyle (right) differ greatly. The differences between chimpanzees and people living close to nature are similar to those between people living close to nature and US citizens. (Modified after Moeller et al. 2014. © Scorpio Verlag in Europa Verlage GmbH, München. Reproduced with permission)

not make a good fit with us, because they are unable to master the interaction with the intestine and the immune and nervous system as well as the long-serving cooperative partners of humans do. Therefore, the dialogue between our "Stone Age intestine" and the "modern" microbiome stutters, and inflammatory diseases are the result. Apparently, we now have a pronounced deficiency of bacteria that calm our immune system, so that susceptible people easily suffer from allergies and other inflammatory diseases. If we were to turn back our diet and lifestyle a bit, and thus create the basis of life for a microbiome that fits better with us, much would be gained.

How Bacteria Alter Their Host

Remote Controlled: An Example from the World of Parasites

From the perspective of commensal bacteria, a host must offer fantastic opportunities! An environment that provides protection, warmth, and a constant supply of food, and all they have to do is treat their host correctly. However, the inhabitants would have to avoid catching their host on the wrong foot and calling his immune response into action, otherwise the plan would not work. Really clever bacteria could be trusted to do even more—they could control their host in such a way that the host fulfills their needs. An example: Wouldn't it be clever of gut bacteria, which are specialized in certain plant fibers, to ignite a craving in us for, say, bananas? If banana fibers then arrived in the intestine, these bacteria would have their ideal food. The production of a substance that increases the desire for bananas would thus be a selection advantage for the species and would lead to it being able to assert itself against competitors. The remotely controlled host would have helped the clever bacteria species into the saddle against their own will.

Since microbiome research is still in its early stages, there are no known examples of a real, bacteria-induced behavior that benefits our inhabitants. However, it is known that our gut flora influences the moods and behavior of their hosts, including their appetite (De Wouters et al. 2021). There are, however, numerous examples from other areas of biology of the extent to which evolution has equipped inhabitants with the ability to specifically influence their hosts. Therefore, I would like to digress from bacteria and introduce a parasite of animals that is a master of manipulation, able to dramatically change the behavior of its host to its own advantage. Perhaps commensal bacteria have similarly advanced, yet undiscovered, abilities to influence their host. As I said: The following example is only intended to illustrate the potential of evolution—whether such abilities will ever be discovered in bacteria, the future must show.

In search of an interesting topic for my diploma thesis as a biologist, I came across the "small liver fluke", a parasitic worm about 1 cm long, which was to shape my professional career. I found this worm and the biology of similar creatures so fascinating that parasitology later became my field of work.

The parasite that captivated me (its Latin name is Dicrocoelium dendriticum) lives as a sexual animal in the bile ducts of the liver of sheep and other herbivors and feeds there on cells and mucus. Its eggs are excreted with the host's feces and then have to be eaten by a very specific type of snail, in which the larvae of the worm grow. Since sheep do not eat snails, the small liver fluke evolved a sophisticated strategy to guide its offspring into the next sheep: It uses ants, whose behavior it manipulates, as a ferry.

To hijack this ferry, the parasite larvae leave their host snail in batches of several dozens early in the morning, at the beginning of the ant rush hour. These little worms are highly attractive to ants and are gladly eaten by the patrolling early risers. Most of them migrate to the abdomen of their new host, while a single larva targets the ant's brain and settles in a very specific area. There, it waits until the siblings in the abdomen have further developed and surrounded themselves with a protective shell. After about a month, the "brain worm" then becomes active and reprograms the behavior of the ant.

While normal ants return to the nest in the evening, the infected insects, as it gets cooler, climb plants near the nest and remain there by biting into the plants. Their jaws cramp so much that the ants can only let go of the plant when the temperatures rise again the next morning. This ensures that, in the early morning hours, just in time for the sheep's breakfast, the fresh green is garnished with infected ants. Thus, the brain worm drives its host ant to suicide, as it is digested by the sheep with the food. In contrast, the parasite larvae pass through the sheep's stomach thanks to their protective shell, colonize the liver and develop into sexual animals. This completes the life cycle of the parasite (Lucius et al. 2017).

This remotely controlled ant is one of the most convincing examples of how extensively inhabitants can reprogram their host. The control of the ant-zombies is fabulously precise: the brain worm always sits in the same brain region and ensures that the ants offer themselves to the sheep for food in time. So far, it is completely unknown how the brain worm locates its target area, precisely intervenes in the brain metabolism of its ant host and then switches on the alternative behavior program when its siblings in the ant's abdomen are ready to travel.

But this is not about the "how". The important thing about this example is that the parasite has developed an incredibly precise mechanism, through the pressure of evolution, for controlling the host. With similarly sophisticated mechanisms, commensal bacteria, which have evolved with humans over millions of years, could manipulate the immune system of their host. With very specifically acting metabolic products, they could, for example, inhibit inflammatory reactions, and thus bring about a harmonious coexistence with their host.

Fat or Thin: A Question of the Microbiome?

"Does the microbiome influence its host?"—this was the topic that drove the science after we learned about the complexity of our inner ecosystem in the 2010s. Jeffrey Gordon, from Washington University in St. Louis, MO, USA, stimulated the scientific discussion in 2013 with a study whose results clearly showed that body weight and microbiome are connected (Ridaura et al. 2013, Fig. 4.8). Demonstrating the influence of bacteria on body weight was a brilliant move: Almost every adult pays attention to their figure sooner or later, and besides, pounds are something tangible. Everyone knows what it means to gain a kilogram, whereas a change of a metabolic parameter is quite abstract for most people. Moreover, the topic is of utmost importance because of the obesity epidemic, with its increased risk for metabolic and inflammatory diseases.

For their study, Gordon and his colleagues had chosen an approach that was based on a combination of human and mouse studies. They first identified a pair of identical twin sisters, one of whom was of normal weight, while the other suffered from obesity. Since identical twins are genetically identical, differences in genetic makeup were ruled out as the cause of the weight differences, and so the researchers focused on the microbiome. To do this, they used the fact that many bacteria of the human gut flora can also thrive in the mouse's gut if there is no competition from local bacteria. This allows the transfer gut bacteria from humans to mice that were either raised sterile or treated with broad-spectrum antibiotics. The empty gut of the recipient animals can also harbor bacteria that would have no chance against the existing gut flora under normal circumstances. The effects of this gut colonization on weight, behavior, immune responses, and other parameters are then observed in comparison with control groups.

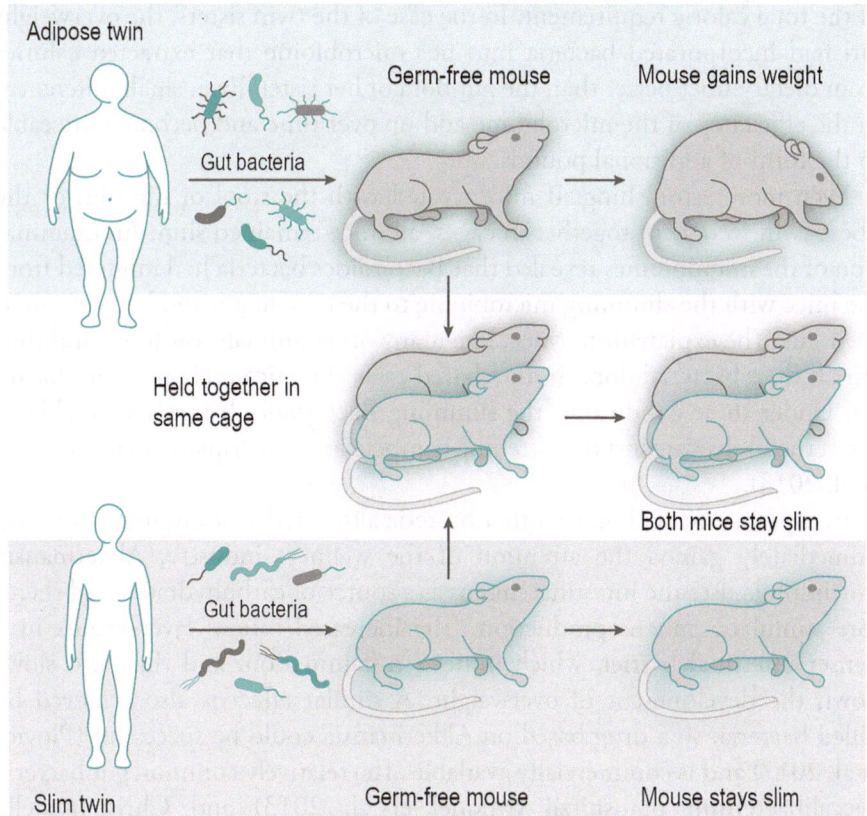

Fig. 4.8 Influence of the microbiome on the body weight of mice in experiments by Ridaura et al. (2013). The transfer of the gut flora of a fat twin to germ-free mice led to weight gain, while the gut flora of a slim twin did not have this effect. When mice were kept together, the gut flora of the slim twin dominated, and the mice remained slim. (Modified after Gerard 2016. © Scorpio Verlag in Europa Verlage GmbH, München. Reproduced with permission)

When the researchers transferred the gut flora of the two sisters to germ-free mice, whose food was rich in dietary fibers, they found, to their surprise, significant effects on the body weight of the rodents. The mice that had been given bacteria from the obese twin developed overweight! Their gut bacteria could break down the dietary fiber and provided their host with additional calories. In contrast, the animals with the microbiome of the slim twin did not gain weight, because their bacteria utilized the dietary fiber in the food less efficiently. So, the body weight depends on, among other things, the microbiome! There are now also numerous studies in humans that confirm these results. It is known that the gut flora provides, on average, about 10%

of the total calorie requirement. In the case of the twin sisters, the overweight girl had incorporated bacteria into her microbiome that extracted calories from dietary fiber better than the gut flora of her sister. Even small differences in the efficiency of the microbiome add up over time and become noticeable in the form of additional pounds.

Even more astonishing: If mice treated with the stool of the slim or the obese twin were kept together in cages, all mice remained slim. An examination of the microbiomes revealed that Bacteroides bacteria had migrated from the mice with the slimming microbiome to the cage mates and had colonized their gut. The explanation: Mice, like many other animals, eat feces, and thus enrich their bacterial flora. In the shared cage, the mice exchanged gut bacteria. Under these conditions, the slimming Bacteroides bacteria were able to assert themselves against the fattening competition and displace them (Ridaura et al. 2013).

In experiments with mice, other bacteria also acted as slimming agents and immediately gained the attention of the wellness industry: Akkermansia muciniphila uses the intestinal mucus as a source of carbohydrates, and therefore stimulates mucus production. The increased mucus layer results in a denser intestinal barrier, which inhibits inflammation, and thus also slows down the development of overweight. A similar effect is also achieved by killed bacteria, so a drug based on Akkermansia could be successful (Plovier et al. 2017) and is commercially available. The relatively common gut bacteria Faecalibacterium prausnitzii (Miquel et al. 2013) and Christensenella (Goodrich et al. 2014) also have a comparable health-promoting effect. However, despite their interesting properties, such probiotic bacteria should be treated with caution, as some lead a double life: If they are not sufficiently supplied with dietary fibers, they can attack the intestinal mucus too much, so that the intestinal barrier suffers and the tendency towards inflammation and susceptibility to infections increases (Desai et al. 2016).

The opposite effect, namely, overweight due to a single type of bacteria, was shown by the Chinese researchers Fei and Zhao from Jiao Tong University in Shanghai. In one of their patients, who suffered from morbid obesity, the gut microbiome consisted of 35% Enterobacter cloacae bacteria, which thrive well on a high-fat diet. This species is otherwise only present in lower densities. Was there a connection between the microbiome and overweight? To find out, the researchers colonized the gut of germ-free mice with Enterobacter bacteria from the obese patient. And indeed: When fed a very high-fat diet, the animals of the experimental group gained much more weight than the control group. Presumably, Enterobacter cloacae triggered inflammatory processes that, in turn, promoted obesity (Fei and Zhao 2013). The bacteria donor, by the way, lost 51 kg of the 175 kg he had previously weighed after his bacteria were deprived of their basis for life by switching the patient to a plant-based and traditional Chinese diet. The bacterial fattening agents were no longer detectable in his stool.

These studies show that the gut flora can influence body weight through the efficiency of food utilization and by influencing inflammatory processes. Fat deposits then, in turn, have an inflammatory effect, as fat cells produce inflammatory cytokines, the adipokines. The fat stored in the abdominal cavity (the "visceral fat") has a particularly fatal effect. This is not the belly fat mocked as "life belt", but fat tissue that accumulates around the intestine. Anyone who carries a lot of this visceral fat has a stronger tendency towards inflammatory reactions due to the adipokines, apart of the other health risks that obesity causes.

However, one should not attribute too much responsibility for body weight to the microbiome. The intestine itself has no fixed upper limit in terms of food intake and takes up whatever easily accessible nutrients are available. The sheer amount of food and its calorie content are therefore crucial for waist size. Those who like to feast on sugar- and fat-rich food without moving much are particularly likely to get a bill for the excess calories in the form of fat deposits. Those who eat moderately, cultivate a slimming microbiome through healthy nutrition and exercise a lot will have less trouble with additional kilos.

Gut Bacteria Also Control Behavior

Not only the weight, but also the behavior of mice is determined by the gut flora. One of the groundbreaking observations on this question comes from neuroscientist Premysl Bercik and his team at MacMaster University in Ontario (Canada). The researchers used inbred mouse strains that "naturally" show different behavior: BALB/c mice are rather anxious and not particularly sociable; let's call them "shy" mice. In contrast, animals of the NIH-Swiss strain are relatively curious and love social contact; they could be described as "cheerful" mice.

If shy or cheerful mice were treated with broad-spectrum antibiotics, the composition of their microbiomes changed—unsurprisingly. At the same time, however, the typical behavioral pattern of the mouse strains reversed for several weeks: the shy mice became cheerful, and the cheerful mice became reserved. As the effect of the antibiotic wore off and the gut flora regenerated after several months, the altered behavior also normalized (Bercik et al. 2011).

Bercik and his colleagues then tested, through bacteria transfer, whether the microbiome was responsible for the changes. They transferred gut bacteria from shy to cheerful mice, which had previously had their own microbiome removed by antibiotics, and vice versa. The recipient mice then demonstrated the behavior typical for the donor animals: While the formerly shy mice, who had had the gut flora of the cheerful animals transferred into them, became more daring, the formerly cheerful mice became more anxious and demonstrated depression-like behaviors after the bacteria transfer. Further experiments could prove that the effect of the transplanted microbiome was not based on nerve signals, nor on altered immune reactions, but on the metabolic products of bacteria. This behavior typical for the mouse strains was therefore determined by the intestinal bacteria!

Meanwhile, there are numerous such experiments that point in the same direction: The microbiome influences the basic psychological moods of mice through different mechanisms. And even more: Treatment with a single strain of bacteria was even able to significantly improve depressive behavior and autism-like disorders in the mouse model, a sensational result! (Hsiao et al. 2013). The reason: The stimulation of the intestinal epithelial cells by the bacteria led to a denser closure of the intestinal barrier, so that certain harmful metabolic products of the bacteria did not enter the bloodstream. Since similar effects have also been demonstrated in humans (e.g., Pinto-Sanches et al. 2017), there have been numerous attempts to treat depression and autism-like disorders, which are becoming increasingly common in the USA, by administering certain lactobacilli, bifidobacteria or Bacteroides species. Meanwhile, the term "psychobiotics" has been coined for this new class of psychoactive remedies (Sarkar et al. 2016). Anyone who wants to learn more about these effects of the microbiome on the psyche should definitely read "The Second Brain" by Emeran Mayer (2016).

Microbial Danger Signals Train Immune Tolerance

If commensal bacteria can influence the weight and behavior of their hosts, it should be easy to believe that they can also interfere with the immune system. Indeed, bacteria—by design, so to speak—act as an alarm signal for the immune system, because as soon as the body senses bacteria-typical molecules, it triggers its inflammation machinery to ward off pathogens. Bacteria, viruses, and fungi are so distantly related to humans that some of their components are completely different from our components. As mentioned earlier: They could be described as molecular trademarks of microbes. The presence of such molecules means potential danger, even if only harmless bacteria are involved.

Such danger signals include surface molecules, but also components of bacterial flagella and certain DNA sequences. By the way, some of the bodies' own substances, which are released in case of injuries, also act as danger signals and stimulate inflammatory responses. Such molecules are sensed by cells of the innate immune system—the simple, but very efficient part of the immune system that we share with insects. They immediately initiate an inflammation by attracting other immune cells and activating them for attack to eliminate the supposed intruders.

Even if harmless bacteria damage the mucus layer and get too close to the intestinal epithelium, the innate immune system is activated. However, it becomes really dangerous when bacteria break through the intestinal barrier and multiply in the abdominal cavity or in the blood. Then, the immune system switches to the highest alarm level and triggers a reaction cascade, the "septic shock", which often ends fatally. Bacteria and the immune system are therefore inherently as incompatible as fire and water. The presence of trillions of potentially dangerous inhabitants inside us is actually playing with fire, a ticking time bomb in the stomach.

One of the most important danger signals is the bacterial lipopolysaccharide (LPS) mentioned earlier in connection with E. coli, a component of the outer membrane of many bacteria. Even in the tiniest amounts, this substance strongly stimulates immune cells. Generations of immunologists have researched this molecule from E. coli and its effect on the immune system. LPS can be detected almost everywhere: in the soil, in drinking water, in food. It is also contained in dust, and wherever there are dense bacterial accumulations, the substance is inevitably present in large quantities, so that it is inhaled. LPS is also produced by many intestinal bacteria, so that the intestinal mucosa is constantly exposed to this substance. However—and this is important to know—not all LPS is the same, because the cell wall molecule of other bacterial species can be less stimulating than that of E. coli and its close relatives. If human contact with such a common and potent stimulator always led to an overactivation of immune cells, our immune system would constantly run amok, and the collateral damage would be immense. Fortunately, efficient mechanisms limit the effects of LPS and even contribute to the development of immune tolerance.

With LPS, it is observed that immune cells react very strongly to first contact with the molecule; afterwards, however, the reaction is at least blocked for a while. The immune system is thus impregnated against further disturbances by contact with the bacterial danger signal, so that it does not derail when subsequently exposed to larger amounts of LPS. Small amounts of the damaging substance thus stimulate regulatory mechanisms and protect against strong stress. Bart Lambrecht and Hamida Hammad from the Belgian University of Ghent compare the process to the adjustment of a set screw, which reduces sensitivity with repeated contact with LPS. Their research group identified a crucial piece of this inflammation inhibition by repeatedly letting mice inhale small doses of LPS and measuring their reaction. On single contact, LPS triggered an inflammation of the lung as expected, but with repeated treatment, the reaction was absent and an enzyme was formed that blocked the transmission of the "danger in delay" information within the cells. Interestingly, the key enzyme A20 not only made the lungs insensitive to LPS, but also simultaneously to other immunological stimuli. Thus, mice with intact A20 enzyme did not develop asthma when exposed to allergy-causing substances. However, if the mice lacked the enzyme, the inflammation inhibition could not be switched on, and asthma developed (Schuijs et al. 2015). Through the A20 mechanism, the otherwise harmful, inflammation-promoting bacterial danger signals thus train immune tolerance!

In humans, too, the A20 enzyme plays an important role, as children with a defect in the corresponding gene cannot regulate the set screw and have—just like the mice lacking the enzyme—an increased probability of suffering from allergies (Schuijs et al. 2015). A similar adjustment of immune responses probably also works in the intestine and impregnates the intestinal cells against foreign stimuli. Frequent contact with bacteria can therefore desensitize! In this context, the popular wisdom "dirt does not hurt" (in German "Dreck macht Speck") makes sense.

Inflammation-Inhibiting or: Stimulating Bacteria

In addition to the bacterial danger signals, which are determined by the blueprint of our inhabitants, there are also a multitude of other molecules that affect the host. For example, many different degradation products are produced during metabolism, and the bacterial cell wall also contains effective substances that inhibit inflammatory responses. To analyze their interaction with the immune system, bacteria strains from humans were transferred to germ-free mice, similar to the studies on weight regulation, and the effects on the mouse's immune system were examined. This approach was used, for example, by the team of Dennis Kasper from the Harvard Medical School in Boston in a groundbreaking study (Geva-Zatorsky et al. 2017). For this, the researchers isolated 53 bacterial strains from the human intestine, colonized the intestine of germ-free mice with them, and characterized their immune cells. The results showed that about a third of the bacterial strains in the mice promoted the development of regulatory T cells (Tregs), which downregulate inflammatory responses with their inhibitory cytokines. The Tregs are key elements of immune tolerance. Interestingly, the inflammation brake could be pressed by very different types of bacteria, so it was not only operated by a certain group of relatives. The ability to inhibit the immune system is therefore widespread among peaceful intestinal inhabitants. Some of the inhibitory components have already been characterized more closely at the molecular level. For example, several Bacteroides species contain a polysaccharide that promotes the development of regulatory T cells in cell cultures and induces the production of the inhibitory cytokine IL-10 (Neff et al. 2016). It can be assumed that such intestinal bacteria, which inhibit inflammatory responses, have proven particularly successful as commensals in the course of evolution.

How relevant the inhibitory bacteria in the intestine are is shown by various diseases. Strong inflammatory activity in patients is usually associated with lower densities of inflammation-inhibiting bacteria. Even in the case of COVID-19 infections, this connection existed, as a comparison of the microbiomes of patients with different clinical symptoms showed. People with pronounced clinical symptoms, which are very much caused by inflammatory responses, had very low densities of inflammation-inhibiting intestinal bacteria. In contrast, patients with mild symptoms had higher densities and healthy people had the highest densities. The inflammation inhibitors in the intestine belong to the usual suspects: In this case, they were Bifidobacteria, Faecalibacterium prausnitzii and Eubacterium rectale (Zuo et al. 2020; Yeoh et al. 2021; Moreira-Rosario et al. 2021). The researchers suspect that, in the case of COVID-19 infections, the intestinal inhabitants mitigate the patients' inflammatory responses, which would otherwise lead to a potentially deadly cytokine storm. In another study, which still needs to be confirmed by independent review, it was found that severe symptoms and deaths from COVID-19 infections coincide with the occurrence of the inflammation-promoting bacterium Enterococcus faecalis in the intestinal microbiome (Ward et al. 2021). These findings suggest that the microbiome can be used prognostically to identify individuals with a particularly high risk early on.

While many commensal bacteria dampen the immune system and calm the intestine, there are also inhabitants who have the opposite effect: They heat up the host's immune response. In mice, it was observed that certain intestinal bacteria, the "segmented filamentous bacteria" (SFBs), sit directly on the surface of intestinal cells and even penetrate somewhat into the cell interior. These bacteria program intestinal epithelial cells and immune cells for an increased defense against pathogens. They activate the cells of the epithelium in such a way that they move closer together and form an even denser closure. This makes the intestinal wall even more impermeable to pathogens. In addition, they activate the mouse's immune system in such a way that very aggressive immune responses are initiated. These Th17-type responses keep pathogenic bacteria in check in the intestine and on other mucous membranes.

To the researchers' surprise, the effect of the SFBs in the intestine even extended to the animals' lungs: There, certain pathogens causing pneumonia were very sustainably decimated by immune responses. However, this activation of the immune system by bacteria in the intestine comes at a price, as, in mice, SFB bacteria can enhance existing autoimmune responses (Schnupf et al. 2017). In humans, closely related bacteria have also been found, and it is suspected that they too can initiate aggressive immune responses that have their advantages and disadvantages. Interestingly, these SFBs in animals and humans are the only known bacteria that the host allows to have such close contact with its own cells without triggering massive defense reactions. It is also noteworthy that they only occur in young animals. It could well be that these commensals are important in the early phase of life for calibrating the immune system.

Probiotics

Can't we quickly and thoroughly change our microbiome with very targeted methods to be healthier overall and also reduce the risk of inflammatory diseases? How about a morning cocktail of bacteria that colonize the gut, push back pathogens, keep the immune system in balance, and also deliver a few valuable vitamins? Advertising suggests that "probiotics", beneficial microorganisms, have this effect. According to a definition by the WHO, these are living microorganisms that have a health benefit for the host when administered in appropriate amounts. So, a variety of products can adorn themselves with the name "probiotic".

A good example of a probiotic bacterium is "E. coli Nissle 1917", which was described more than 100 years ago and is still approved as a medicine for the treatment of chronic intestinal inflammations and diarrhea in infants and toddlers. The history of the oldest probiotic on the market also reflects the development of bacteriology: At the beginning of the twentieth century, before the dawn of the age of antibiotics, researchers tried to combat bacterial pathogens with other bacteria. It had been observed that, in mixed bacterial cultures, under certain conditions, one species prevailed over the others.

Couldn't this effect be used to limit harmful bacteria? The young physician Alfred Nissle, head of the Baden Medical Examination Office for Infectious Diseases in Freiburg, analyzed the stool of patients suffering from diarrheal diseases with this thought in mind.

For this purpose, stool samples were suspended and small amounts of them were spread on agar plates to cultivate bacteria. In most of the cultures that Nissle examined, the diarrhea pathogens had prevailed after some time and overgrown other bacteria. However, in rare cases, E. coli bacteria had gained the upper hand and displaced the diarrhea pathogens. In 1917, during the First World War, Nissle isolated such an E. coli strain from the stool of a non-commissioned officer. The soldier had served in the Balkans, where a diarrhea epidemic was raging among his comrades at the time, but he had remained healthy. Nissle suspected that his gut bacteria had protected the soldier against diarrhea, and it turned out he was right. Thus, the strain E. coli Nissle 1917, which is the correct designation today, turned out to be a multi-talent in the course of time.

E. coli Nissle 1917 not only kills salmonella and other related diarrhea pathogens, but also has a pronounced anti-inflammatory effect. Researchers later observed that immune cells release anti-inflammatory messengers under the influence of the Nissle bacterium, and thus calm their environment. In addition, the tiny organism causes a denser closure of the intestinal barrier, strengthens the resistance of epithelial cells against the penetration by pathogens, and boosts the antibody response in the gut. These properties are not unusual for a successful gut bacterium, which has to defend itself against competitors and dampen the host's immune responses in order to live in peace with it. However, while the variety of positive effects of E. coli Nissle 1917 is impressive, perhaps it will turn out in the future that other gut bacteria also have similar abilities.

The promises by advertising that probiotics help with intestinal complaints and other ailments are not wrong, but, unfortunately, do not always apply for everyone and sometimes not at all, because probiotics work, as to be expected, very differently and individually. In humans, the newly introduced bacteria meet an ecosystem of hundreds of bacterial species, into which they must integrate if the success is to be sustainable. Therefore, it is difficult to prove the healing effect with the strict standards applied to medications, and the official evaluations often turn out to be very restrained. A typical example is a statement by the German Federal Institute for Risk Assessment on probiotics in infant nutrition: "Infant foods enriched with probiotics are therefore no better suited for the nutrition of healthy infants than products without probiotics" (BfR 2015). In plain language, this means that the benefit of probiotics could not be proven. Thus, probiotics were long ridiculed by conventional medicine, but they enjoy a high status in alternative medicine and the nutrition scene.

A treatment with probiotics can improve the condition if, for example, one is frequently sick and suffers from infections of the throat, nose, ears or urinary tract. Thus, children who had consumed probiotic drinks in studies were 24% less likely to suffer from intestinal infections (Merenstein et al. 2010) and a meta-analysis showed an effectiveness of probiotics against colds (Hao et al. 2015). Probiotic preparations are also used to recolonize the intestines after treatment with antibiotics or to prevent allergies and neurodermatitis. But not only can infections, diarrhea and constipation be influenced by probiotics, so can brain activity and the psyche, thus clever sales strategists created the new term "psychobiotics" (Bermudez-Humaram 2019).

The idea that bacteria could be health-promoting originally came from the immunologist Illja Illjitsch Metschnikow, who received the Nobel Prize for Medicine in 1908. On his travels in Bulgaria, he noticed that a lot of yogurt was eaten there and that many people reached an impressively high age. He postulated, in 1907, that the yogurt bacteria only recently discovered were the cause of longevity, without having any evidence for this. For him, the colon was basically a harmful organ in which putrefactive bacteria lead to self-poisoning. The "good" yogurt bacteria would kill these harmful bacteria with the lactic acid they produce, and thus prolong life, he theorized. This hypothesis, which was pulled out of thin air, led to yogurt still being considered a kind of panacea in some circles today.

Yogurt is a good example of a probiotic food. The origin of such foods is probably due to the fact that microorganisms extend the shelf life of dairy products and other foods through "fermentation". In this process, the microbes break down substances in the absence of oxygen and gain energy to multiply. Their metabolic products, such as lactic acid, keep competing molds and bacteria at bay. This is how yogurt, sour milk, kefir and many types of cheese are made, as well as sauerkraut and fermented bean products. Probiotic drinks like kombucha and kvass are also made by fermenting them with live microbes.

In addition to the longer shelf life, another positive effect of the microorganisms is significant: By breaking down carbohydrates, foods become more digestible. For example, yogurt and hard cheese are more tolerable for people with lactose intolerance because the milk sugar was broken down by bacteria. Often, flavoring substances are also formed during fermentation; just think of a Camembert, with its delicate aroma, which is due to mold. However, the actual probiotic effect is mostly based on the living microbes that enter the intestine with the food, multiply there for at least a while and produce favorable metabolites. Yet, the vast majority do not survive the acid bath of the stomach passage, so one should not be too impressed by the immense numbers of bacteria that some yogurt brands advertise.

For the fermentation of food, very different types of bacteria and fungi are used more or less deliberately. In many cases, certain strains of lactic acid bacteria (Lactococcus or Lactobacillus species) are used as starter cultures, their name referring to the lactic acid they give off as a metabolic product. Since lactic acid bacteria are almost everywhere in the environment, untargeted fermentation is anything but complicated: For example, to make sauerkraut, you shred white cabbage, pound it to break down the cells, layer it in an airtight container and cover it with brine. If the surface is covered so that oxygen has no access, but the resulting $CO2$ can escape, the lactic acid bacteria adhering to the cabbage leaves multiply massively. The lactic acid they produce acidifies the liquid so strongly that other microbes have no chance. When, after a few weeks, the lactic acid has reached such a high concentration that even the lactic acid bacteria can no longer multiply, the sauerkraut is ready. However, the probiotic effect of sauerkraut is lost during cooking, because the positive effects are achieved only with living bacteria that colonize the intestine.

The industry offers the opportunity to enrich the inner ecosystem very specifically with probiotic preparations. Pharmaceutical probiotics usually consist of freeze-dried bacteria or certain yeasts. They are usually administered in capsules that release their contents in the intestine. This means that, compared to probiotic foods, there is a better chance from the outset that large numbers of bacteria will reach the intestine, which increases the likelihood of colonization. In addition to lactobacilli and bifidobacteria, strepto- and enterococci species and certain E. coli strains are used as probiotics. Also, yeasts of the species Saccharomyces boulardi are approved for the treatment of diarrhea. Some manufacturers increase the chance that bacteria will establish themselves in the intestine for a longer period of time by filling their intestinal capsules with several different strains. Occasionally, along with the bacteria, a "prebiotic", i.e., a suitable dietary fiber, is also administered in the intestinal capsule. The idea is to give the newcomers a head start. Even if the amount of dietary fiber provided is very small, such measures are effective in advertising, especially when the combination of probiotic and prebiotic is then marketed as a "synbiotic".

Those who study the package inserts of probiotic preparations will find almost exclusively well-known bacterial species that have been used for generations for the production of fermented foods or as medicines listed there. However, one searches in vain for microbes, which have only recently been described and should be particularly suitable as anti-inflammatory agents, because they break down dietary fiber into short-chain fatty acids or stabilize the intestinal barrier. This one-sided orientation is due to legal regulations that, since 1978, have required very costly testing procedures for the new approval of pharmaceuticals. This involves clinical studies proving their safety and efficacy, which would cost millions of euros for the approval of new probiotics.

On the other hand, microbes that have proven to be harmless in the past, and are therefore classified as "GRAS" (generally regarded as safe), can be registered using a simplified procedure. Manufacturers who want to avoid risky investments therefore rely on already known bacteria or fungi. It will be interesting to see when a new generation of probiotics with a wider range of effects comes onto the market. Bacteria like Faecalibacterium prausnitzii, Akkermansia muciniphila, Roseburia and Christensenella are attractive candidates. However, oxygen is toxic to these useful inhabitants, so that administration in capsules or as powder requires development work. Moreover, such new probiotics still have to pass the tests for efficacy and safety.

The Molecular Code of the Inflammation Brake

Every gut bacterium that a human carries is comparable to a tiny chemical factory that constantly releases a variety of substances in its exhaust plume. However, it does not work like a chemical plant in earlier times, crudely, with distillation plants or boilers with high pressure and high temperatures, but rather in an energy-saving manner, using molecular machines, the enzymes. With this arsenal of bacterial enzymes, our inhabitants process the food residues that were not digested in the small intestine. As a result, thousands of different metabolic products, known as "metabolites", are produced. Often, such substances form the basis of life for other bacterial species, which further degrade them and produce additional metabolites in the process. Many of these substances penetrate the intestinal wall, spill into the blood, circulate in the body and have an effect on the metabolism and the immune and nervous systems. If the bacteria disappear, for example, as a result of antibiotic treatment or a change in diet, the effect quickly decreases. Some of these metabolites are key molecules for immune tolerance.

A major source of bacterial metabolites is the previously mentioned dietary fiber, i.e., plant structural components, fibers or soluble substances, which are indigestible for humans, but that represent valuable food for many bacteria in the large intestine. This material consists mainly of carbohydrates. However, proteins, fats and plant constituents, such as polyphenols, carotenoids or glucosinolates, are also broken down by bacteria. Many of these substances come from plant cells that pass through the small intestine unharmed because they are surrounded by a solid cell wall, and only in the large intestine are they broken down by bacteria and release their contents. Thus, highly active plant constituents that are formed as a defense against insect grazing or as protection against UV radiation get liberated. Such substances can either act directly or unfold their effects after degradation and conversion by the gut bacteria. Since there are thousands of different plant substances, the variety of resulting metabolites is huge. Even in a small piece of fruit, hundreds of different substances can be detected. Which metabolites humans are exposed to, therefore, depends on their diet, but also on the capacity of their microbiome. Depending on the composition of the gut flora, our inhabitants can produce different metabolites from the same plant substances. As far as their effect is concerned, science is still in its early stages.

The most important metabolites produced by the degradation of plant dietary fiber are the short-chain fatty acids mentioned earlier, such as acetic acid, propionic acid and butyric acid. These small molecules provide energy to intestinal cells and the liver, amounting to about 10% of our total needs, but they are also indispensable as calming pills for the immune system, leading to the formation of regulatory T cells (Fig. 4.6). They also strengthen the integrity of the intestinal barrier.

The Tregs migrate from the intestine to the farthest corner of the body, carrying their calming message with them (Smith et al. 2013; Haghikia et al. 2015). Immune tolerance is not only mediated by Tregs, but also by other immune cells such as neutrophils, macrophages and eosinophils, which respond to various bacterial metabolites and slow down inflammation with cytokines.

Many metabolites of the gut flora have a similar calming effect on the immune system as short-chain fatty acids. Among the better-known substances are secondary bile acids, which are produced during bacterial degradation of components of bile juice (Zeng et al. 2019), but also indoles, i.e., metabolites that are produced during the breakdown of the amino acid tryptophan. Substances derived from food, such as polyphenols, are also important for limiting damage caused by inflammatory responses. This group of substances includes many blue, red, and yellow colors from plants. They can act directly on intestinal cells, but, in many cases, they are further processed by intestinal bacteria into potent metabolites that, as antioxidants, capture highly reactive free radicals, and thus protect the tissue and DNA. Without these inhibitory influences of the microbiome, the immune system would be in a state of constant alarm, triggered by irrelevant signals.

Many of the bacterial metabolites affect the host by binding to a system of sensors with which almost all cells are equipped. Of these antennas, the G-protein-coupled receptors (GPRs), there are over 1000 different variants. They sit on the surface of cells and inform them about the state of the environment. Depending on how they are built and on which cells they sit, they can recognize food molecules, smells, or light, so they are the tongue, the nose, or the eyes of cells. They inform the cell about, among other things, the concentration of metabolic products or the acidity of the fluid in the environment (Robert and Mackay 2018). When bacterial metabolites bind to such GPRs, the stimulus triggers very specific reactions of the corresponding cell. In this way, our body, which is constantly flooded with bacterial metabolic products, is exposed to the influence of the gut flora. Immune cells also have GPRs, so bacterial metabolites can communicate with them to ignite or dampen inflammation.

The Long-Term Programming of Immune Tolerance

The previous sections describe two essential mechanisms of immune tolerance: On the one hand, repeated contact with bacterial danger signals desensitizes immune cells, similar to how the impregnation of an old-fashioned raincoat protects against moisture. This protection is not permanent, because, if the danger signals are absent for a long time, the immune cells become more reactive again. On the other hand, bacterial metabolites, such as short-chain fatty acids, apply an immune brake by initiating the development of Tregs, which inhibit inflammatory responses with their messenger substances. This dampening effect also subsides without constant resupply of the critical bacterial substances.

Beyond these short-term effects, contact with bacterial danger signals and metabolites also shapes the immune system in the long term. With repeated contact with such stimuli, cellular reactions become ingrained and solidify over time. Just as, in cross-country skiing, the first runner sets the track and the others then hardly deviate from it because they can move forward more effortlessly on the groomed track, many reactions of immune cells also follow a pre-established pattern. This also applies to the Tregs, which, thanks to their immunological memory, react more strongly to renewed contact with a known substance than the previous time (Rosenblum et al. 2015). They "learn", so to speak, and write the processes in a cellular program. The cells of the innate immune response are also programmed by repeated contact with microbial danger signals, and their reactions then follow the established pattern. This imprinting does not only refer to individual cells, but also to the cooperation between cell populations, which then follows an established pattern. In this way, the immune system "learns" to respond to a known stimulus with a programmed reaction. Therefore, someone who was desensitized as a toddler through diverse bacterial contact has a low probability of developing allergies in adulthood due to their programming.

The decisive time window for this long-term imprinting can be directly determined in mice: it extends from the time before birth to weaning, when the first solid food is taken. In humans, too, immune programming works best in toddlers. Already in the uterus, the education of the child's immune system begins through microbial products that reach the fetus via the maternal circulation (Ansaldo et al. 2021). A vaginal birth and prolonged breast-feeding of the baby promote the healthy, gradual development of its microbiome, the products of which influence and imprint the regulatory circuits of the child's immune system at an appropriate time. This programming works best in the first 3–6 months of the child's life (Nabhani and Eberl 2020). The imprinting is supported and maintained if continuous contact with a diverse bacterial flora remains in the long term. A good example of this is the protection against inflammatory diseases for children who grow up on traditionally operating farms, with their rich bacterial flora (see the section "The Farm Effect" in Chap. 3). Studies on the effect of antibiotic treatments in newborns suggest the consequences that a disturbed balance between the partners in this important developmental period could have: In children who had been treated with a broad-spectrum antibiotic as newborns due to a threatened sepsis, the microbiome was less diverse up to the age of six, they had a higher body weight, and boys in the treated group were significantly smaller at 6 years than those in the control group (Uzan-Yulzari et al. 2021).

These learning processes of the cell are controlled by epigenetic processes, i.e., cellular mechanisms that facilitate or hinder access to genes without changing their DNA sequence. They can be compared to switches that control the reading of genes. Accordingly, the genes can be read better or worse after activating an epigenetic switch. Epigenetic processes serve to store established reaction patterns of the cell. The more often a stimulus-response chain runs, the more the established track solidifies. Such imprinted patterns can persist for a very long time and can even be passed on from the mother to the child and to subsequent generations. On the other hand, the programming can fade in the absence of stimuli or be broken and overwritten in the event of serious disruptions.

Observations suggest that immune tolerance decreases over time and the tendency towards inflammation increases if the bacterial diversity to which one is exposed through the microbiome and the environment decreases. It is also assumed that strong disturbances of the microbial ecosystem, in which the usual calming signals are absent for a long time, can lead to a loss of programmed immune tolerance. For example, infections that damage the intestinal barrier and cause strong inflammation could overwrite the anchored cellular programs of the immune brake. It is also conceivable that disturbances of the intestinal flora caused by improper antibiotic treatment could change the tolerant milieu of the intestine. Under such circumstances, unfavorable regulatory circuits can then become entrenched, leading to subliminal inflammation and disease. Anyone who wants to prevent this should take care of their microbiome through a healthy diet that provides the bacteria with enough dietary fiber and protective plant substances. Contact with environmental bacteria is also important, as they stimulate the immune system with their danger signals and trigger anti-inflammatory mechanisms. Thus, a diverse bacterial environment consolidates the tolerance mechanisms of the immune system.

Alarm in the Gut

The Gut Flora as a Danger

The cooperation between humans and gut flora usually works inconspicuously, as long as the bacterial species form and maintain a balanced ecosystem overall. However, in inflammatory diseases, certain groups and species of bacteria in the gut are typically over- or underrepresented, and the number of species is reduced. At this point, the chicken-or-egg problem inevitably arises: Did the disturbed bacterial community trigger the disease, or is it a consequence of the disease?

Unfortunately, there are no simple explanatory patterns here, because the triggers of inflammatory diseases are usually multifactorial. Often, defects in the intestinal barrier that can be triggered by bacteria, but can also have completely different causes, play an important role. In this context, multiple external influences such as infections, stress, or—especially in the case of obesity—elevated levels of inflammatory messengers act together on the intestinal barrier. The delicate mucous membrane then becomes permeable, allowing bacteria and their metabolites to come into contact with the immune system and cause inflammation, which, in turn, further damages the intestine. Certain human gene variants that influence the cohesion of cells or the composition of the intestinal mucus can also weaken the intestinal barrier and increase the risk of disease.

Dr. Malin Johansson, an internationally renowned specialist in intestinal diseases from the University of Gothenburg in Sweden, explained to me, with a simple scenario, how even a change in diet can lead to inflammation in the intestine: Many intestinal bacteria, which need plant fibers as food, also graze the top layer of mucus from the surface of the large intestine, which contains carbohydrates and dead epithelial cells, and is therefore nutrient-rich. Normally, the bacteria are prevented from penetrating deeper into the mucus by antimicrobial substances produced by the intestinal epithelial cells. However, if there is a drastic change in diet and not enough dietary fiber is available, the bacteria adapt and become more resistant to the antimicrobial agents. They can then penetrate deeper into the protective layer and eat more mucus. If, under these circumstances, not enough mucus is produced, for example, in people with certain genetic defects, the intestinal barrier no longer functions completely. Bacteria and their products thus come into direct contact with the cells of the intestinal epithelium, which are then stressed and move apart.

Through such gaps in the intestinal barrier, bacteria and their danger signals reach the underlying immune cells. This stimulus triggers an alarm: inflammation occurs and can spread further if the immune response is not downregulated immediately (Desai et al. 2016). More bacteria then penetrate through the defective intestinal barrier and the inflammation intensifies. In the process, cytokines are released that attract and activate even more immune cells and, among other things, also stimulate cells of the enteric nervous system, which transmit the signals to the brain. Other cytokines enter the blood and cause fatigue, fever, and metabolic changes.

Similarly, intestinal inflammation can occur when the intestinal barrier is damaged by pathogens or stress (in the broadest sense). If frequently recurring stimuli repeatedly cause inflammation, the control circuits of the immune system adjust to this state and the inflammation continues without external stimulus, becoming chronic. This situation is dangerous because, in the cauldron of inflammation, immune responses are randomly generated. Normally, the immune system prevents the recognition of self or self-similar molecules, but in inflammation, the control mechanisms can go awry. Then, immune responses against bacterial components can be triggered that also recognize self molecules with a similar molecular structure and attack them. Such "molecular cross-reactions" exist, for example, in rheumatoid arthritis between bacterial molecules and components of the joint cartilage. If the inflammation mechanisms become entrenched, the attack on the body's own tissue continues, even if the originally triggering bacteria have disappeared. Therefore, a defective intestinal barrier promotes the development of autoimmune diseases.

In alternative medicine, many diseases—from inflammatory diseases to digestive disorders, headaches to depressive moods—are attributed to a permeable intestinal barrier. The totality of these ailments is referred to as "Leaky Gut Syndrome". Under this keyword, you can find a lot of information and various treatment suggestions on the internet. Indeed, it makes sense to consider a disturbed intestinal barrier as an important element of many diseases. However, conventional medicine does not accept the syndrome as an independent disease, because, from its point of view, disturbances of the intestinal barrier are not the cause, but rather the result of diseases. In the conceptual framework of conventional medicine, diseases are defined by their cause, because eliminating the primary cause of the disease offers the best chances of healing. Therefore, the treatment should address the causes. In any case, it makes sense to bring the unbalanced microbiome back into balance through healthy nutrition and a lifestyle that includes exercise and a lot of contact with nature. However, it is advisable to also accept the offer of established medicine for diseases that indicate a permeable intestine. Treating persistent intestinal disorders without knowing the cause would be reckless.

"Evil by Nature": Pathogenic Bacteria

In May 2011, the Robert Koch Institute in Berlin, Germany's "epidemic police", reported a suspiciously high number of severe, bloody diarrheal diseases, some with kidney failure, mostly from northern Germany. There were even deaths to mourn. The outbreak quickly became a media event. An epidemic outbreak in Germany! In a country with such a highly developed health system! Enterohemorrhagic E. coli of the strain EHEC O104:H4, as it is technically called, could be isolated from the dying patients. Enterohemorrhagic means that the bacteria cause bleeding by attacking blood vessels with a toxin they produce, causing small veins to leak.

This was the hour of microbiologist Helge Karch. The professor and head of the Hygiene Institute at the University of Münster had specialized in pathogenic bacteria, i.e., disease-causing E. coli, since his doctoral thesis; he knows all the molecular tricks of the pathogens and all the shades of the diseases they cause. His team had the necessary modern diagnostic methods and soon solved the mystery: The epidemic germ was a bacterium that is rare but well known in Germany. It causes hemolytic uremic syndrome (HUS), a disease characterized by severe bleeding and kidney damage. Sequencing of the genome revealed that it was a hybrid of two pathogenic strains, one that was also resistant to certain antibiotics. The bacterium produced several toxins and also had the ability to attach itself to the intestinal epithelium in dense colonies. But why was this pathogen able to cause an epidemic? With its molecular profile, which was now available, the search for the source of the outbreak began, while more and more patients with severe disease symptoms were admitted to hospitals.

Where did these bacteria come from? The epidemic detectives of the Robert Koch Institute took up the trail, mapped the cases, interviewed the sick, checked suspicious sources, and traced delivery routes. The majority of the sick were women; another commonality was a preference for tomatoes, cucumbers, and salads. Five weeks after the start of the outbreak, a probable source had finally been found: a horticultural business from Lower Saxony that produced tasty sprouts from fenugreek seeds imported from Egypt. These sprouts, which are added to salads, were probably contaminated. The pattern of disease outbreaks matched the delivery routes of this delicacy exactly. However, there was no final confirmation of the suspicion, as no samples containing EHEC bacteria were found. The business was closed and, by the end of June, the epidemic had subsided. Ultimately, however, it is not clear whether the danger has been averted once and for all. Professor Helge Karch is not sure about this. The Ärzteblatt of May 3, 2016, quotes him: "The strain O104:H4 still exists, but it has not caused any more outbreaks and is rare, a rarity." How did this outbreak, during which over 4000 people fell ill and 53 patients died, occur? What made this pathogen so aggressive? These questions remain open.

Our commensal bacteria in the gut could be compared to a herd of peaceful sheep that stay obediently in their pasture and are content with the available food, as long as the fences, i.e., the intestinal barrier, are intact. This existence is modest, but, as a commensal bacterium, one can survive well in the long term. But what if a few particularly clever comrades suddenly realize that the meager food is not enough for them, and they destroy the barrier with brute force to open up additional food sources? Such attacks occur when pathogenic bacteria spread. Often, they are relatives of commensal bacteria that have taken over genes from other species, and thus acquired new abilities with which they ruthlessly exploit and damage the host. Sometimes, it is only a few additional genes that turn a commensal bacterium from a promoter of health into a pathogen, sometimes whole gene packages.

One common faction of these "pathogenicity factors" is toxins, such as the hemolytic EHEC toxin, which destroys host tissue, and thus releases nutrients for the pathogenic bacteria. Other toxins act as a nerve poison, such as the wrinkle iron "Botox", a deadly poison from Botulinum bacteria that kill their host to multiply in the decomposing carcass. Other gene packages enable bacteria to inject molecules into host cells with needle-like structures that reprogram the cell. Such a modified cell then takes the bacterium into its interior, where it can multiply—protected from immune responses. Thanks to acquired genes, bacteria can also form, for example, short, filamentous structures, the pili, with which they attach themselves to the intestinal epithelium, so that they are not washed away by the peristalsis.

Even with such sophisticated pathogenicity factors, it is not necessarily easy for pathogens to conquer a host. The typical pathogenic bacteria of the intestine reach their destination, for example, with contaminated food or polluted water. However, if only a few aggressive germs are introduced, they often have no chance against the established intestinal flora.

The resident bacteria keep the surfaces densely populated, fight for the food with the invaders, and confront them with antibacterial molecules. This defense against pathogens is one of the most important tasks of the microbiome (Kamada et al. 2012). However, if the infection dose is very high, the pathogens' chances of breaching the ranks of the resident bacteria and establishing themselves increase. Therefore, the danger posed by pathogens is always also a question of dose. A few dozen salmonella can be easily handled, while, for example, a spoiled egg salad, in which billions of diarrhea pathogens are present, is quite likely to give one roaring diarrhea. Even stress, antibiotic treatment, altered diet or other changes can disrupt the balance, disturbing the intestinal flora and allowing pathogens to spread.

Many pathogenic bacteria reliably live in small numbers as unobtrusive members of the bacterial community in the gut. In healthy individuals, they are kept in check by the commensal gut bacteria and the immune system. However, disturbances in the species composition in the gut offer these so-called opportunists the chance to multiply massively, allowing them to, for example, attack the intestinal epithelium, leading to severe diarrhea. In hospitals, these opportunistic pathogens particularly endanger immunocompromised and elderly people. Particularly feared in such situations is Clostridium difficile, a bacterium that can cause severe, bloody diarrhea. C. diff., as the medical abbreviation goes, is found in the gut of 2–5% of healthy individuals, but in nursing homes, it is found in up to 50% of residents. Most of the time, the bacterium behaves inconspicuously, but it can prevail in a gut with destabilized bacterial flora. If the corresponding strain is antibiotic-resistant, very determined action must be taken to prevent fatal disease courses. Then, the best therapy is a re-colonization of the gut through fecal transplantation, in which the complete microbiome of a healthy person is transferred (see also the excursus "Fecal Transplantation" in Chap. 8). With this method, infections with Clostridium difficile have been cured in over 90% of cases.

Antibiotics, a Double-Edged Sword

Antibiotics have a bad reputation: They are found in chicken, are ineffective for colds, and breed resistant pathogens. However, it is easy to forget what humanity owes to these drugs: Thanks to antibiotics, many previously fatal infections in industrialized countries have become a trivial matter. However, these wonder weapons have a significant limitation: They only work against bacteria, not against viruses and parasites. Therefore, for the treatment of influenza, AIDS, COVID-19 or malaria, we are dependent on other, sometimes still very inadequate, drugs. Thanks to antibiotics and hygiene, only 1–5% of deaths in the industrialized world today are due to infectious diseases, while, in some developing countries, it is still over 40%. If you live in one of the less developed countries in Africa, the risk of dying from an infection is about ten times as high as in Central Europe.

Antibiotics are essential for the treatment of certain infections, but they can also kill useful bacteria as collateral damage. Therefore, the excessive use of systemic—i.e., affecting the entire body—antibiotics causes damage to the microbiome that is often still underestimated today. Orally administered antibiotics often cause a real clear-cutting in the gut. After discontinuing the antibiotics, the bacterial flora usually regenerates, but the species composition can shift or species that previously led a marginal existence may not survive the clear-cutting and die out. Therefore, repeated intake of antibiotics leads to permanent changes in the species spectrum of the microbiome and reduces the species diversity in the gut (Palleja et al. 2018). Especially in toddlers up to the third year of life, disturbances of the microbiome due to antibiotic treatment lead to an increased risk of allergic diseases and chronic intestinal inflammation later in life.

If you research the consequences of antibiotic treatment, another clear connection inevitably emerges: Quite obviously, repeated treatment with systemic antibiotics leads to increased weight gain! Shortly after penicillin, the discovery of Alexander Fleming, was brought to market in the post-war years, antibiotics were even used as "performance enhancers" in animal fattening. The use of antibiotics in chicken fattening was observed to increase weight gain by 50% and in cattle by 20%. The effect was attributed to the promotion of growth-enhancement and the inhibition of harmful intestinal bacteria.

Bacterial species that could extract many calories from food and make them accessible to the animal were considered beneficial. The newly discovered antibiotics were seen as turbo drugs that acted like a kind of cheap fertilizer that was added to the feed to achieve better growth and, at the same time, prevent infections. Since 2006, the use of antibiotics as growth promoters in the EU has been banned, but the drugs can still be used in animal production to treat infections, and therefore still have a wide distribution.

Antibiotics have a similar effect in humans: As early as 1955, the physicians Thomas Haight and William Pierce reported, in the Journal of Nutrition, on a study with 310 recruits from the American Navy who were divided into three groups and then had to swallow Aureomycin, Penicillin or a placebo daily for 7 weeks. After this "cure", those treated with antibiotics had gained an average of 2.0 kg, but the placebo recipients only gained 1.2 kg. The difference was only 800 g, which may seem insignificant, but, in comparison, the antibiotics had increased weight gain by 67%! No wonder, then, that antibiotics came to be seen as strengthening drugs, and were thus administered to malnourished children in the USA, for example. Especially in children up to 3 years of age and with repeated administration, various antibiotics lead to increased weight gain in later life. Even with short-term use and at low doses, the drugs have this effect (Cox and Blaser 2015; Del Fiol et al. 2018). At the same time that antibiotic use increased, the obesity epidemic began, a development that—starting in the USA—was to plague the Western world in the coming years. A temporal coincidence does not yet mean that two events are causally related, but an overwhelming number of indications suggest that the improper use of antibiotics contributes to the immense spread of overweight, which, in turn, contributes to the increase in inflammatory diseases.

Another pressing problem of medicine is related to antibiotics: Bacterial pathogens that are resistant to antibiotics are increasingly appearing, especially in hospitals. Such resistances are particularly likely to develop in treatments with insufficiently large doses of antibiotics, allowing some resistant bacteria to survive and spread. Through horizontal gene transfer, their protective genes can then be passed on to other bacterial species. This is how resistant bacteria are constantly created in animal fattening, especially in chicken production, through the use of antibiotics, said bacteria then also entering humans through contaminated food. Some of these germs, such as the notorious multi-resistant pus pathogen Staphylococcus aureus (MRSA), can be transmitted from animals to humans. The usual antibiotics are ineffective against the infections they cause. For example, in German clinics, animal breeders are screened separately before admission, because they are potential carriers of MRSA. After all, they could bring the dangerous germs into the clinic, where immunocompromised people would be helplessly exposed to them. Through the massive use of antibiotics, humans have effectively disarmed themselves: antibiotic-resistant bacteria are rapidly increasing, and the chapter of bacterial infections, thought to have ended, continues as multi-resistant germs take the place of the classic pathogens.

The use of systemically acting antibiotics is therefore far from trivial, as even short-term applications disrupt the sensitive balance of the microbiome. The consequences—increased risk of inflammatory diseases, obesity, and the production of resistant pathogens—underline how important the balance of our inner ecosystem is.

References

Amurugam M et al (2011) Enterotypes of the human gut microbiome. Nature 437:174–180

Ansaldo E, Farley TK, Belkaid Y (2021) Control of immunity by microbiota. Ann Rev Immunol 39:449–479

Bercik P et al (2011) The intestinal microbiota affect central levels of brain-derived neurotropic factor and behavior in mice. Gastroenterol 141:599–609

Bermudez-Humaram LG (2019) From probiotics to psychobiotics: live beneficial bacteria which act on the brain-gut axis. Nutrients 11:890

BfR (2015) Announcement No. 025/2015 from 14.8.2015: Infant starter and follow-on nutrition: Health benefits of probiotic bacteria are not proven

Blaser M (2017) The theory of the disappearing microbiota. Nat Rev Immunol 17:461–463

Browning KN et al (2017) Vagus nerve in appetite regulation, mood and intestinal inflammation. Gastroenterol 152:730–744

Carrera-Bastos P et al (2011) The Western diet and lifestyle and diseases of civilization. Res Rep Clin Cardiol 2:15–35

Clemente JC et al (2015) The microbiome of uncontacted Amerindians. Sci Adv 1:e1500183

Cox LM, Blaser MJ (2015) Antibiotics in early life and obesity. Nat Rev Endocrinol 11:182–190

David LA et al (2014) Diet rapidly and reproducibly alters the human gut microbiome. Nature 505:559–563

De Andres J et al (2017) Physiological translocation of lactic acid bacteria during pregnancy contributes to the composition of the milk microbiota in mice. Nutrients 10:14

De Filippo C et al (2010) Impact of diet in shaping gut microbiota revealed by a comparative study in children from Europe and rural Africa. PNAS 107:14691–14696

De Wouters A et al (2021) Gut microbes participate in food preference alterations during obesity. Gut Microbes 13:1959242

Del Fiol FS et al (2018) Obesity: a new adverse effect of antibiotics? Front Pharmacol 9:1408

Desai MS et al (2016) A dietary fiber-deprived gut microbiota degrades the colonic mucus barrier and enhances pathogen susceptibility. Cell 167:1339–1353

El Kaoutary A et al (2013) The abundance and variety of carbohydrate-active enzymes in the human gut microbiota. Nat Rev Microbiol 11:497–504

Fei N, Zhao L (2013) An opportunistic pathogen isolated from the gut of an obese human causes obesity in germfree mice. ISME J 7:880–884

Feretti P et al (2018) Mother-to-infant microbial transmission from different body sites shapes the developing infant gut microbiome. Cell Host Microbe 24:133–145

Fragiadakis GK et al (2019) Links between environment, diet, and the hunter-gatherer microbiome. Gut Microbes 10:216–227

Gensollen T et al (2016) How colonization by microbiota in early life shapes the immune system. Science 352:539–543

Gerard P (2016) Obesity due to gut flora. In: Microbiome. Compact spectrum. Spectrum Publishing, Heidelberg

Geva-Zatorsky N et al (2017) Mining the human gut microbiota for immunomodulatory organisms. Cell 168:928–943

Gilbert JA et al (2018) Current understanding of the human microbiome. Nat Med 24:392–400

Gonzales F et al (2021) Distinct changes occur in the human breast milk microbiome between early and established lactation in breast-feeding Guatemalan mothers. Front Microbiol 12:557180

Goodrich JK et al (2014) Human genetics shape the gut microbiome. Cell 159:789–799

Gurven M, Kaplan H (2007) Longevity among hunter-gatherers: a cross-cultural examination. Popul Dev Res 33:321–365

Haghikia A et al (2015) Dietary fatty acids impact central nervous autoimmunity via the small intestine. Immunity 43:817–829

Hao Q et al (2015) Probiotics for preventing acute upper respiratory tract infections. Cochrane Database Syst Rev 3:CD006895

Hehemann JH et al (2010) Transfer of carbohydrate-active enzymes from marine bacteria to Japanese gut microbiota. Nature 464:908–912

Helander HF, Fändricks L (2014) Surface area of the digestive tract – revisited. Scand J Gastroenterol 49:681–689

Hsiao EY et al (2013) Microbiota modulate behavioral and physiological abnormalities associated with neurodevelopmental disorders. Cell 155:1451–1463

Kamada N et al (2012) Regulated virulence controls the ability of a pathogen to compete with the gut microbiota. Science 336:1325–1329

Kim KS et al (2016) Dietary antigens limit mucosal immunity by inducing regulatory T cells in the small intestine. Science 351:858–863

Koeth R et al (2019) L-carnitine in omnivorous diets induces an atherogenic gut microbial pathway in humans. J Clin Invest 129:373–387

Louca S et al (2019) A census-based estimate of Earth's bacterial and archaeal diversity. PLoS Biol 17:e3000106

Lucius R et al (2017) The biology of parasites. Wiley VCH, Weinheim

Maier L et al (2018) Extensive impact of non-antibiotic drugs on human gut bacteria. Nature 555:327–628

Man WH et al (2017) The microbiota of the respiratory tract: gatekeeper to respiratory health. Nat Rev Microbiol 15:259–270

Mayer EA (2016) The mind-gut connection: how the astonishing dialogue taking place in our bodies impacts health, weight, and mood. Harper Collins

Merenstein D et al (2010) Use of a fermented dairy probiotic drink containing lactobacillus casei (DN-114001) to decrease the rate of illness in kids: the DRINK study. A patient-oriented, double-blind cluster-randomized, placebo-controlled, clinical trial. Eur J Clin Nutr 64:669–677

Mittrücker HW et al (2016) Lack of microbiota reduces innate responses and enhances adaptive immunity against listeria monocytogenes infection. Eur J Immunol 44:1710–1715

Miquel S et al (2013) Faecalibacterium prausnitzii and human intestinal health. Current Opinion Microbiol 16:255–261

Miquel S et al (2014) Ecology and metabolism of the beneficial intestinal commensal bacterium Faecalibacterium prausnitzii. Gut microbes 5:146–151

Moeller AH et al (2014) Rapid changes in the gut microbiome during human evolution. PNAS 111:16431–16435

Moeller AH et al (2016) Cospeciation of gut microbiota with hominids. Science 353:380–383

Moeller AH et al (2017) The shrinking human gut microbiome. Curr Opin Microbiol 38:30–35

Moreira-Rosario A et al (2021) Gut microbiota diversity and C-reactive protein are predictors of disease severity in COVID-19 patients. Front Microbiol 12:705020

Mukopadhya I et al (2018) Sporulation capability and amylosome conservation among human colonic and rumen isolates of the keystone starch degrader Ruminococcus bromii. Environ Microbiol 20:324–336

Nabhani ZA, Eberl G (2020) Imprinting of the immune system by the microbiota early in life. Mucosal Immunol 13:183–189

Nayak RR et al (2021) Methotrexate impacts conserved pathways in diverse human gut bacteria leading to decreases in host immune activation. Cell Host Microbe 29:362–377

Neff CP et al (2016) Diverse intestinal bacteria contain putative zwitterionic capsular polysaccharides with antiinflammatory properties. Cell Host Microbe 20:535–547

O'Keefe SJ (2019) The association between dietary fibre deficiency and high-income lifestyle-associated diseases. Burkitt's hypothesis revisited. Lancet Gastroenterol Hepatol 4:994–996

Obregon-Tito A et al (2015) Subsistence strategies in traditional societies distinguish gut microbiomes. Nat Commun 6:6505

Palleja A et al (2018) Recovery of gut microbiota of healthy adults following antibiotic exposure. Nat Microbiol 3:1255–1265

Pasolli P et al (2019) Extensive unexplored human microbiome diversity revealed over 150 000 genomes from metagenomes spanning age, geography, and lifestyle. Cell 176:649–662

Pinto-Sanchez MI et al (2017) Probiotic Bifidobacterium longum NCC3001 reduces depression scores and alters brain activity: a pilot study in patients with irritable bowel syndrome. Gastroenterol 153:448–459

Plovier H et al (2017) A purified membrane protein from Akkermansia muciniphila or the pasteurized bacterium improves metabolism in obese and diabetic mice. Nat Med 23:107–113

Porter NT et al (2018) Bacteroides thetaiotaomicron. Trends Microbiol 26:966–967

Rajilic-Stojanovic M et al (2015) Intestinal microbiota and diet in IBS: causes, consequences, or epiphenomena? Am J Gastroenterol 110:278–287

Ridaura VK et al (2013) Gut microbiota from twins discordant for obesity modulate metabolism in mice. Science 341:1079

Rinninella E et al (2019) What is a healthy gut microbiota composition? A changing ecosystem across age, environment, diet and diseases. Microorganisms 7:14

Robert R, Mackay CR (2018) Gas-coupled GPCRs GPR65 and GPR174. Downers for immune responses. Immunol Cell Biol 96:341–343

Rodriguez JM et al (2021) The gut-breast axis: programming health for life. Nutrients 13:606

Rodriguez-Sillke Y et al (2021) Recognition of food antigens by the mucosal and systemic immune system. Consequences for intestinal development and homeostasis. Int J Med Microbiol 311:151493

Rosenblum MD et al (2015) Regulatory T cell memory. Nat Rev Immunol 16:90–101

Saei AA, Barzegari A (2012) The microbiome: the forgotten organ of the astronaut's body–probiotics beyond terrestrial limits. Future Microbiol 7:1037–1046

Sarkar A et al (2016) Psychobiotics and the manipulation of bacteria-gut-brain signals. Trends Neurosci 39:763–781

Schnupf P et al (2017) Segmented filamentous bacteria, Th 17 inducers and helpers in a hostile world. Curr Opin Microbiol 35:100–109

Schuijs MJ et al (2015) Farm dust and endotoxin protects against allergy through A20 induction in lung epithelial cells. Science 349:1106–1110

Sender R et al (2016) Revised estimates for the number of human and bacteria cells in the body. PLoS Biol 14:e1002533

Sevelsted A et al (2015) Cesarean section and chronic immune disorders. Pediatrics 135:e92–e98

Smith PM et al (2013) The microbial metabolites, short-chain fatty acids, regulate colonic Treg homeostasis. Science 341:569–573

Sommer F, Bäckhed F (2013) The gut microbiota – masters of host development and physiology. Nat Rev Microbiol 11:227–238

Song SJ et al (2013) Cohabitating family members share microbiota with one another and with their dogs. elife 2:e00458

Sun J et al (2020) Environmental remodeling of human gut microbiota and antibiotic resistome in livestock farms. Nat Commun 11:1427

Tazume S et al (1991) Effects of germfree status and food restriction on longevity and growth of mice. Exp Anim 40:517–522

Tett A et al (2021) Prevotella diversity, niches and interactions with the human host. Nat Rev Microbiol 19:585–599

Thorburn AN et al (2014) Diet, metabolites, and "western-lifestyle" inflammatory diseases. Immunity 40:833–842

Turroni F et al (2014) Molecular dialogue between the human gut microbiota and the host: a lactobacillus and Bifidobacterium perspective. Cell Mol Life Sci 71:183–203

Uzan-Yulzari A et al (2021) Neonatal antibiotic exposure impairs child growth during the first six years of life by perturbing intestinal microbial colonization. Nat Commun 12:443

Vangay P et al (2018) US immigration westernizes the human gut microbiome. Cell 175:962–972

Visekruna A et al (2019) Intestinal development and homeostasis require activation and apoptosis of diet-reactive T cells. J Clin Invest 129:1972–1983

Wagenaar CA et al (2021) The effect of dietary interventions on chronic inflammatory diseases in relation to the microbiome: a systematic review. Nutrients 13:3208

Wang G et al (2019) Bridging intestinal immunity and gut microbiota by metabolites. Cell Mol Life Sci 76:3917–3937

Ward DV et al (2021) The intestinal and oral microbiomes are robust predictors of COVID-19 severity and the main predictor of COVID-19-related fatality. https://doi.org/10.1101/2021.01.05.20249061

Waters JL, Ley RE (2019) The human gut bacteria Christensenellaceae are widespread, heritable and associated with health. BMC Biol 17:83

Weiner HL et al (2011) Oral Tolerance. Immunol Rev 241:241–259

Wibowo MC et al (2021) Reconstruction of ancient microbial genomes from the human gut. Nature 594:235

Yatsunenko T et al (2012) human gut microbiome viewed across age and geography. Nature 486:222–228

Yeoh YK et al (2021) Gut microbiota composition reflects disease severity and dysfunctional immune responses in patients with COVID-19. Gut 70:698–706

Zeißig S (2016) Die physiologische Standortflora. In: Stallmach A, Vehreschild MJGT (eds) Mikrobiom – Wissensstand und Perspektiven. Walter de Gruyter GmbH, Berlin/Boston

Zeng H et al (2019) Secondary bile acids and short chain fatty acids in the colon: a focus on colonic microbiome, cell proliferation, inflammation, and cancer. Int J Mol Sci 20:1214

Zhao L et al (2019) Adaptive evolution within gut microbiomes of healthy people. Cell Host Microbe 25:656–667

Zipperer A et al (2016) Human commensals producing a novel antibiotic impair pathogen colonization. Nature 535:511–516

Zuo T et al (2020) Alterations in gut microbiota of patients with COVID-19 during time of hospitalization. Gastroenterol 159:944–955

5

Inflammatory Diseases

Contents

Allergic Diseases

Allergic diseases can have very different manifestations, as hay fever, asthma, food allergy, or atopic dermatitis. These diseases share the following mechanism: Involving antibodies, a foreign stimulus leads to the rapid activation of cells that initiate an inflammatory response. Allergic diseases are an example of immune responses that have gone awry. The Western lifestyle has led to a massive increase in such diseases since the 1960s. Originally, allergic reactions were directed against parasites, but these pests hardly play a role for us anymore. Thus, in our modern society, they no longer serve any biological purpose.

Allergies, As Almost Everyone Knows Them: Itching, Sneezing, Coughing

Almost everyone has had experience with minor allergic reactions. A typical example is mosquito bites: As soon as the insect has taken off again after a brief visit, a strongly itching wheal develops within minutes, usually subsiding after some time. Without this defense, the bloodsuckers could feast much longer. Similar mechanisms are also active in the intestine and keep parasitic worms in check. However, allergy sufferers also react to molecules from plants and animals that are similar to parasite proteins (Tyagi et al. 2015). Such allergies can affect the entire body and lead to the most severe reactions, up to and including death. In technical terms, allergic diseases are referred to as "atopies" (from Greek: a topos = without place, as they are not limited to a specific organ).

In industrial societies, allergic diseases are the most common chronic diseases (EAACI 2018), while they are rare in societies living close to nature. The best-known are the classic allergies, such as hay fever or food allergies, but also allergic asthma and atopic dermatitis (Latin: skin inflammation). In Germany, according to the Robert Koch Institute, more than 40% of adults have either experienced an allergic disease at some point or are still suffering from it (Bergmann et al. 2016). The European Society for Immunology suspects that, in the not-too-distant future, more than half of the population will be allergic (EAACI 2018). However, in recent years in some industrialized countries, the number of new cases has not continued to rise, while the epidemic in emerging and developing countries continues to gain momentum.

The tendency to allergies is partly genetically determined, but the increase in allergic diseases is attributed to the western lifestyle. Particularly important for the development of allergic diseases is early childhood: Already in the womb, but also in the first years of life, the still plastic immune system receives decisive impulses from products of commensal bacteria, which cause long-term programming (Ansaldo 2021). Children who were exposed to a diverse microbial flora through their microbiome and environment tend to have balanced immune responses, while children without these stimuli have a higher risk of allergies. In a Swedish study, city children were about eight times more likely to develop allergies than children who grew up on farms. Caesarean section births also significantly increase the risk of allergic diseases in children, because they have a disturbed microbiome due to the lack of contact with maternal bacteria. Similarly, bottle-fed children are more likely to develop allergies later in life than children who were breastfed for at least 6 months (Haspeslagh et al. 2018).

Along with early imprinting, the composition of the microbiome also plays an important role. Children with allergies have fewer bacteria with anti-inflammatory properties such as Bifidobacteria, Faecalibacterium, and Akkermansia (Fujimori et al. 2016) and fewer short-chain fatty acids (Roduit et al. 2018) in their stool.

Atopy occurs when the immune system reacts to substances that are actually harmless, such as pollen, animal hair, house dust, or certain food components, which penetrate through the protective barrier of the mucous membrane or skin. The substances that cause allergies are called allergens. In classic allergies, the mucous membranes of the nose and intestines are typical entry points for allergens; in the case of atopic dermatitis, it is the skin. The first contact with an allergen goes unnoticed and leads to sensitization in susceptible individuals, i.e., the formation of a certain class of antibodies, the IgE anti-bodies. These antibodies attach themselves to the surface of certain cells, the mast cells, which are located in the mucous membranes or the skin. Just as a hedgehog is covered with spikes, these cells are studded with protruding IgE antibodies. The antibodies act as sensors for the very specific allergen they recognize. Such IgE-equipped mast cells become active immediately when their IgE sensors report an allergen. Within seconds, they release a mix of molecules that make the walls of small blood vessels and tissues permeable and attract inflammatory cells. These inflammatory cells then release toxic substances that are actually supposed to repel bloodsuckers or ward off para-sitic worms, but also damage the body's own tissue (Fig. 5.1).

Allergic reactions are among the most sensitive biological reactions known. An IgE-equipped mast cell can release its products when only two antibodies sitting on its surface bind a single allergen molecule. This means that, even in

A   First exposure to allergen

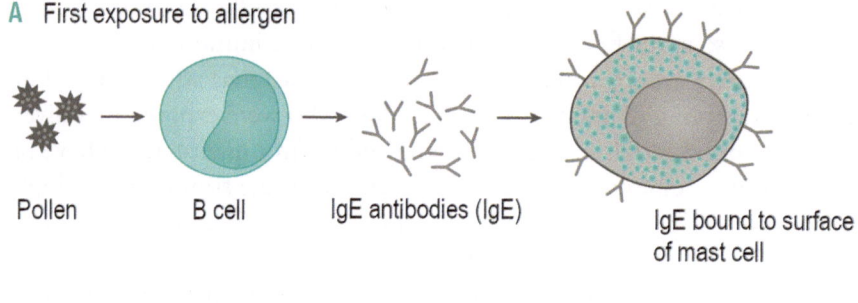

Pollen   B cell   IgE antibodies (IgE)   IgE bound to surface of mast cell

B   Further exposures to allergen

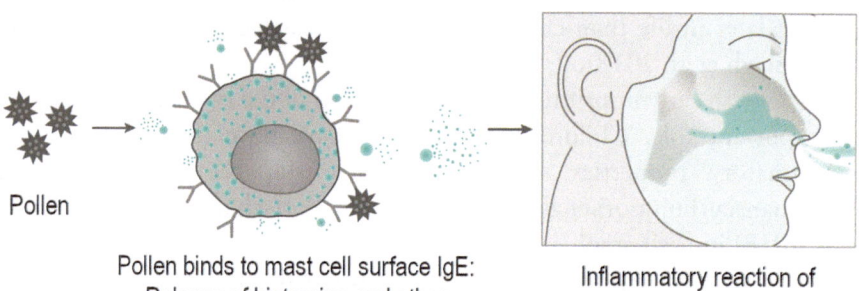

Pollen

Pollen binds to mast cell surface IgE: Release of histamine and other substances

Inflammatory reaction of the mucous membrane

Fig. 5.1 Development of hay fever. (**a**) Upon first contact with pollen, B cells produce IgE antibodies that bind to the surface of mast cells. (**b**) Upon further contact, pollen components bind to these IgE antibodies; the mast cells release histamine and other substances that initiate inflammation. (© Scorpio Verlag in Europa Verlage GmbH, München. Reproduced with permission)

unimaginably low dilution, allergens can trigger a reaction, which explains the enormous sensitivity of allergy sufferers. Usually, the symptoms of allergic diseases are limited to itchy skin areas, swollen mucous membranes, watery eyes, and spasmodic cough. However, allergies can also trigger a potentially fatal chain reaction leading to an "anaphylactic shock". In this case, an exaggerated reaction causes blood pressure to drop, unconsciousness to occur, and the person to fall into a coma.

Hay Fever

In hay fever, allergens from pollen, cat hair, or other substances irritate the mucous membranes of the upper respiratory tract and the eyes. Most reactions are highly specific to a particular allergen, such as pollen from ryegrass, but not necessarily other grasses. Some people "collect" additional allergies over the course of their allergic "career"; for example, if they were initially only allergic to guinea pig hair, they may later also react to hair from mice, dogs, and cats. The consequences are sneezing, swelling of the nasal mucous membranes, watery eyes, and conjunctivitis. This is often accompanied by a general feeling of fatigue.

Allergies that started as hay fever can, over time, also affect the lower respiratory tract and develop into bronchial asthma. According to the pollen calendar, those affected can calculate when they will be out of action: In January, allergies to hazelnut begin, later, pollen from Trees and grasses make life difficult for allergy sufferers, and towards autumn, nettles and ragweed are the culprits.

As already described in detail in the introductory chapter, hay fever was hardly known in the past, but is now so commonplace that it is often taken for granted. In Germany, one in seven adults and one in ten children (Bergmann et al. 2016) suffer from it, but significantly more people have IgE antibodies against allergens, and are thus sensitized, so that an allergy can break out in them when (previously unknown) triggering factors act. Medications can alleviate the symptoms, but cannot cure the cause of the allergy. Anyone who wants to tackle the problem at its root must undergo hyposensitization. In this process, a doctor injects the allergen to which the allergic person reacts under the skin. The injections have to be given repeatedly over a longer time span, usually 3 years. When the immune system is confronted with the allergen in this way, it often reacts differently compared to the contact with the mucous membrane and is reprogrammed. It now produces a different, harmless type of immune response, and allergic reactions cease, even when allergens hit the mucous membranes of the nose and eyes.

Allergic Asthma

The incidence of asthma has also increased dramatically in recent decades. The disease is caused by allergic and inflammatory reactions of the bronchi and lungs. Asthma was hardly mentioned in pediatric textbooks in the 1960s, but then began to appear more and more frequently in statistics in the 1980s. However, this increase was not really noticed until the 1990s (Platts-Mills 2015). When a large study with Finnish recruits found a continuous, dramatic increase in the prevalence of asthma, alarm bells rang: Between 1966 and 1989, there had been a more than 20-fold increase in Finland (Haahtela et al. 1990). Compared to 1966, about six times more conscripts had to be declared unfit for service due to asthma in 1989. Asthma seemed to question the Finns' fitness for military service! These figures could no longer be ignored. Asthma had finally arrived in the consciousness of the Finns, but also in the scientific world.

The differences in the frequency of asthma between Western lifestyle countries and developing countries are striking: According to a World Health Study initiated by the WHO in 2002, typically, between 3% and 4% of the people surveyed in African countries had suffered from asthma in the previous 12 months. In countries with high prevalence, such as Australia, Sweden and Great Britain, the rates were around 20% (To et al. 2012).

The immune responses in asthma follow the basic pattern of allergic reactions. However, the IgE-occupied mast cells, which attract inflammatory cells upon allergen contact, are located in the lower respiratory tract. The finely branched lung airways, the bronchi and bronchioles, also try to expel the allergens by producing mucus and contracting spasmodically. This leads to severe and long-lasting coughing, with shortness of breath. The attracted inflammatory cells accumulate in large quantities near the airways and can also migrate into the airways themselves. They release aggressive substances that damage the tissue. If the allergen stimulus disappears, for example, because the pollen season is over, these inflammations can recede. This asthma caused by allergens is referred to as extrinsic, i.e., caused by external stimuli, asthma.

If, on the other hand, contact with the allergen persists for a long time, the inflammations of the airways do not recede, because immunological circuits have become established: The inflammations become chronic. The walls of the airways thicken and narrow. The inflammatory cells are in a constant state of alarm, and even the smallest amounts of the allergen now trigger severe coughing fits. This lowers the threshold for an asthma attack so much that, eventually, stimuli such as air pollutants, certain medications, cold or stress—i.e., not just the allergen originally responsible—can act as triggers. The reaction chain can become self-sustaining, running completely independently of the original allergy. This is then referred to as intrinsic, i.e., caused by internal stimuli, asthma. Smoking is a factor that massively promotes the development from extrinsic to intrinsic asthma.

Food Allergies

The most common triggers of food allergies are milk, chicken eggs, peanuts and nuts, soy, wheat, fish and shellfish. In total, there are over 800 substances with known allergenic effects. Food allergies frequently occur in early childhood, but often decrease over time, so that they have disappeared around the time of puberty. The reactions occur within minutes to hours after contact with the allergen. Common reactions are skin reactions, such as hives, which means, more or less, large wheals, severe itching, redness and skin swelling. Similar processes can occur in the mucous membranes. This can lead to sneezing, coughing and mucus in the respiratory tract. The tongue can swell, and there can be nausea, diarrhea, flatulence and vomiting. The most severe allergic manifestation is anaphylactic shock, which can even lead to death due to circulatory collapse. Because of the frequency with which food allergy sufferers are exposed to dangers, restaurants in Germany are required to list allergens from 14 main groups that are contained in the dishes offered.

The country with the highest rates of food allergies is Australia, where about 10% of all children are affected. In Germany around 2010, between 2% and 3% of adults were allergic to at least one food, while in children, a frequency of about 4% was assumed (Langen et al. 2013). However, many more people believe they suffer from a food allergy. These are often, in fact, intolerances, which manifest similarly to allergies, but occur without the involvement of IgE.

In the case of a food allergy, the avoidance of the corresponding allergen is currently recommended in Germany. So, if you are allergic to peanuts, you should avoid all peanut products. What seems difficult, but still somewhat possible, with peanuts is really hard when it comes to allergies to milk components, wheat or soy. Many of these products are contained as hidden additives or as contamination in small amounts in food. Another problem is cross-allergies, i.e., related plants or animals that have very similar allergens. For example, in the case of a celery allergy, eating carrots can also trigger an attack. Only some allergens are destroyed by cooking, while others are largely heat-stable, for example, certain allergens from fish.

But how do you avoid the development of a food allergy? Here, science has made a 180-degree turn and recognized that the immune system of toddlers is tolerized by contact with potential allergens. The prime example of this connection is peanut allergy. As recently as 2000, parents in the USA were advised to prevent peanut allergy by withholding peanuts and peanut-containing products from their children from the outset. The frequency of this allergy then continued to increase, instead of, as expected, decreasing, until the course was reversed. The decisive factor was studies that showed that British children had a ten times higher risk of peanut allergy compared to Israeli children (Du Toit et al. 2008). The assumption: The little Brits did not get to eat peanut products as toddlers, so their immune system was unprepared when it encountered the allergens later. In contrast, peanut products were a staple part of the diet for Israeli babies aged 8–14 months. This was a strong indication of tolerance induction through early contact with the allergen.

Controlled studies confirmed this suspicion (Du Toit et al. 2015). Early contact with allergens thus protects against later disease! The food industry has taken this lesson to heart and has scaled back the production of allergen-free baby food. Since fetuses in the womb are also exposed to immunological feedback loops, they too benefit from the mothers' tolerance, and the children develop fewer allergies later. Therefore, German allergologists no longer recommend avoiding potential food allergens during pregnancy (DGAKI/ DGKJ 2014).

Atopic Dermatitis

Atopic dermatitis, also known as atopic eczema or neurodermatitis, occurs as an inflammatory skin disease, particularly in children (Weidiger and Novak 2016). The occurrence of the disease has increased significantly worldwide since the 1960s, although, in recent years, there has been no further increase in many industrialized countries (Williams et al. 2016). In Germany, about 13.2% of children and 3.5% of adults are affected (Bergmann et al. 2016), in the USA, the disease is significantly more common, affecting 7–10% in adults.

The disease most commonly affects toddlers from the third month onwards. It then manifests itself in reddened, inflamed skin, predominantly on the cheeks, on the face or over the entirety of the head, including under the hair. Crusts form, often referred to as milk scabs, because they look dark like burnt milk. In about 50% of children with atopic dermatitis, the disorder has disappeared by the age of 4. Even after that, the frequency continues to decrease, but the disease can persist into adulthood. Then, the insides of the elbows, the backs of the knees, the face, and the neck are mainly affected by itching, weeping rashes. Even if the atopic dermatitis disappears, there is often a tendency towards other allergic diseases. Atopic dermatitis is a heavy burden: sufferers cannot concentrate and do not get enough sleep, so they are less efficient in their endeavors. In addition, the eczema is often disfiguring, causing the afflicted to feel socially excluded.

Healthy skin is covered by a protective film of water, salts, fats, and sebum gland secretions, and is thus protected from drying out. In addition, a multitude of bacteria and fungi frolic on the skin without it leading to disease. However, if the supply of fat is insufficient or the cells of the skin surface do not form a dense seal due to a genetic predisposition, the skin dries out and becomes cracked, allowing foreign substances and germs to gain access.

People who suffer from such skin problems and a tendency towards allergies have a high risk for atopic dermatitis. When bacteria or fungi penetrate their skin, IgE antibodies are formed. An allergic inflammation is set in motion that further irritates the skin. The itching leads to scratching, which creates new entry points for foreign substances and pathogens. The tissue fluid that is also released is a breeding ground for bacteria, such as staphylococci, which then penetrate the wounds and provoke further immune responses. This creates a vicious circle that is difficult to break. The disease occurs in bouts of varying duration and intensity; the course is influenced by diet, stress, and other factors. In some variants of atopic dermatitis, autoimmune responses are also involved in the reaction, so that the disease can persist even when the original triggers are removed.

Since there is no causative therapy for treating atopic dermatitis, one must try to influence the course by avoiding allergens, engaging in very good skin care and availing oneself of anti-allergic therapies. If bacteria and fungi play an important role as triggers, the doctor will also prescribe antibiotics or antifungals. Interestingly, atopic dermatitis can often be influenced by diet. Thus, avoiding sugar, acidic fruit (for example, citrus fruits) and glutamine-containing foods (for example, hard cheese, smoked meat, red wine, legumes) can bring about a significant improvement.

Recommended for Imitation: The Finnish Allergy Program

In 2012, about 10% of the adult population of Finland was medically diagnosed with asthma (Jousilahti et al. 2016), while, in 1966, it had only been 0.29% (Haahtela et al. 1990). These figures show a 35-fold increase within 40 years! Besides asthma, allergies and atopic dermatitis have also increased significantly. Finland is thus one of the most affected countries in the world.

Comparative studies show that this increase was triggered by the western lifestyle. A prime example of this is the studies in Karelia presented in the third chapter: This region is divided between Finland and Russia, the population is genetically very similar, and climate, vegetation and other factors are identical. On the Finnish side, the prevalence of allergic diseases reaches record levels, while it is very low on the Russian side (Haahtela et al. 2015). There, the people still grow up under poor conditions and the standard of living is still much lower than in the Finnish part of Karelia.

From these studies, the Finns have developed very specific insights into the causes of the allergy epidemic, which provide important starting points for the prevention of inflammatory diseases. In a video interview, I spoke with Harri Alenius, a prominent immunologist, who is a professor at the famous Swedish Karolinska Institute in Stockholm and at the University of Helsinki. He explained to me that, according to Finnish data, contact with environmental bacteria significantly influences the immune system and causes tolerization. While the world is very intensively dealing with the influence of the gut microbiome on inflammatory diseases, Finnish researchers have also focused on the bacterial environment of people. They were able to show experimentally, for example, that equipping kindergartens with forest soil and plants led to changes in the microbiome of the children and improved their inflammation values (Roslund et al. 2020, see also Chap. 7 "A New Pact"). They regularly found increased numbers of Gamma-Proteobacteria on the skin, in the dust of apartments, in the soil of playgrounds and on plants in the vicinity of people who are free from allergies and asthma. Therefore, they suspect that these microbes play an important role in the tolerization of people (Hanski et al. 2012; Fyhrquist et al. 2014; Ruokolainen et al. 2015).

In Finland, these findings have been incorporated into a national allergy program that ran from 2008 to 2018 and aimed at preventing and combatting allergic diseases (Haahtela et al. 2012). The program assumed that the cause of allergies, asthma and atopic dermatitis lies in insufficient immune tolerance, which therefore needs to be strengthened. To convey these contents, doctors, medical staff and pharmacy professionals were trained nationwide. In kindergartens and schools, the information was disseminated by organizations and associations.

An important message was not to avoid allergens at the first sign of reactions, as was done in the past. In the case of mild allergic reactions, they rather attempted to achieve tolerization through limited exposure. In other words, for example, in the case of a mild allergic reaction to nuts, it was recommended not to completely eliminate them from the diet, but to continue eating them in small amounts, as this supports tolerance. However, severe diseases, such as asthma attacks, were consistently treated. Contact with the living environment was given great importance. Thus, with a "Go to Nature" program, efforts were made in kindergartens to shift activities more towards nature, to bring children into contact with microbes from soil and plants. As part of these activities, a "Green City" program was also launched to bring more greenery into the inner cities, and thus increase the diversity of microbial stimuli. But there was also an effort to encourage those affected to take a more rational approach to their suffering and to motivate people to self-manage their disease.

This Finnish initiative was very successful and led, for example, to a reduction in hospital admissions due to asthma by almost 90%. It reduced the individual suffering of thousands of patients, relieved the health system (Haahtela et al. 2017), and is thus a model for similar programs in other countries.

Chronic Inflammatory Bowel Disease (IBD)

The Disease IBD

Constantly having to go to the toilet, always tired and worn out, abdominal pain, even at night... a nightmare! About 400,000 people in Germany who suffer from chronic inflammatory bowel disease (IBD) suffer this fate.

In an interview, Britta Siegmund, Professor of Gastroenterology at the Berlin Charité and an internationally known specialist on IBD, explains very vividly how the disease develops. Around 75% of the risk of IBD is due to environmental factors, especially smoking and poor diet, but genetic factors also contribute about 25% of the risk. A typical scenario: Risk genes, which are important in the constant remodeling and repair of damage to the intestinal surface, make the labile balance of the intestine more susceptible to disturbances in those at risk of IBD. If a person at risk with such genetic factors goes on vacation in an unfamiliar environment, the changed diet can throw the intestinal flora out of balance and cause severe traveler's diarrhea, which also attacks the mucus layer of the intestinal surface. Often, an infection with viruses that kill cells of the intestinal mucosa, creating tiny gaps in the epithelium, is added to such a disturbance—because the defense is weakened.

If the repair mechanisms of our digestive tract do not work correctly in this situation, bacteria from the intestinal flora penetrate into the tissues below the intestinal epithelium. There, they encounter immune cells, which are alarmed by the unusual, overwhelming contact with bacteria-typical molecules and attract inflammatory cells. These try to fend off the invaders with aggressive molecules and, in the process, also damage the cell layer of the intestinal epithelium, so that more bacteria penetrate into the tissue, which fuels the turmoil.

This is how inflammation foci develop, which can enlarge and become chronic if the wounds do not heal, and the immune response is not efficiently downregulated. Similar scenarios are conceivable in infections with diarrhea pathogens or after antibiotic treatments, if they lead to massive disturbances of the intestinal flora. Since altered conditions exist in the inflamed intestine, other types of bacteria now thrive, which may further support the inflammation.

There are two different forms, Ulcerative Colitis (UC) and Crohn's Disease (CD), which have many similarities. The disease occurs in bouts, and patients with active disease have severe abdominal pain and diarrhea with bloody-mucous stool. They suffer from stool urgency and intestinal cramps. Going to the toilet 20 times a day is not an exception. In severe disease, fever and weight loss also manifest. Periods of illness are often followed by months-long, quieter phases, which one seeks to extend through treatment with medication.

The cause of IBD is an exaggerated immune response to bacteria in the gut flora, leading to inflammation. IBD is not psychologically or stress-induced, as was previously assumed, and usually occurs between the ages of 20 and 40, often affecting people in the prime of their lives. In many regions, UC occurs about twice as often as CD, the reasons for which are unknown. The disease patterns of UC and CD are different, but overlap to some extent:

Ulcerative Colitis: Here, the inflammation of the mucous membrane is typically limited to the colon, and there to the intestinal surface. It usually starts in the rectum and can extend continuously to the upper section of the colon over years. The symptoms are strongest in patients whose entire colon is chronically inflamed.

Crohn's Disease: Different regions of the entire gastrointestinal tract can be inflamed, from the mouth through the esophagus, the stomach and small intestine to the colon. The small intestine is most often affected. The mucosal inflammations reach deeper into the tissue and also affect the muscle layer, so that scars often form that impair the intestinal function. Abscesses and fistulas easily form, and there can be intestinal constrictions. During operations, there is a risk that the remaining, healthy intestinal sections will become inflamed.

Chronic intestinal inflammations do not remain confined to the intestine in many patients, but affect the entire body over the course of the disease. Thus, 30 years after the first diagnosis, about 50% of those affected suffer from various inflammations, which can cause more severe complaints than the intestinal disease itself. About a third of those affected suffer from joint inflammations (arthritis), eye inflammations and inflammations of the bile ducts, which can lead to liver cirrhosis (Vavricka et al. 2015), but are less common. In addition, IBD patients have a significantly increased risk of colorectal cancer.

The Worldwide Increase in IBD

There have probably always been isolated cases of IBD, but it was not until the second half of the nineteenth century that IBD was defined as a separate disease in England. In 1909, a cohort of 300 patients with diseases that would now be called IBD was presented for the first time at a conference in London. Several decades later, a sharp increase in cases was also noticed in other European countries (Mulder et al. 2014).

Crohn's disease first came into the public eye when US President Dwight D. Eisenhower had to have a 25 cm long piece of small intestine removed in a dramatic operation in 1956. The patient's intestine had become so narrowed by inflammation that it was almost completely blocked, which would have been fatal without immediate surgery. Until then, Crohn's disease was only known to a small circle of specialists. As Der Spiegel wrote in an issue from the time, "American newspapers sought to fathom in column-long speculations how Eisenhower's intestinal inflammation could have arisen". The most important political consequence of Eisenhower's illness was his renunciation of a re-election bid, announced by his personal physician on the night of the operation while the patient was still exhausted and in deep sleep.

Since about 1960, the prevalence of IBD in industrialized countries, especially in North America and Northern Europe, has been steadily increasing.

From 1962 to 2010, the number of new cases (incidence) typically increased five to tenfold in the regions of Europe that were studied (Burisch and Munkholm 2015). In some regions, the curve then flattened, and the frequency of new cases is now stable. However, since IBD is not an immediately fatal disease, the prevalence, i.e., the total number of IBD patients in the population, continues to rise sharply. Currently, in industrialized countries, typically, about 0.5% of the population suffers from IBD. The extent to which IBD is a typical disease of affluent countries becomes clear when looking at a European distribution map (Burisch et al. 2014). In affluent Finland, the IBD rate increased more than threefold from 1987 to 2014 (Virta et al. 2017), leading newspapers to refer to IBD as the "new national disease". In contrast, in the adjacent part of Russia, where the standard of living is much lower, the increase in the IBD rate is much lower.

In many countries of the global South, the disease was hardly known until recently. However, the Asian region has caught up significantly in recent decades (Kaplan 2015; Kedia and Ahuja 2017), and in some countries, the numbers are skyrocketing. Hong Kong, for example, recorded a 30-fold increase in IBD between 1985 and 2014 (Ng et al. 2017), but in absolute numbers, it still lags behind the traditional industrial nations.

Thus, like most other inflammatory diseases, IBD is a typical civilization disease that respects no borders. The increase is attributed to the Western lifestyle. There is disagreement about the significance of individual factors as triggers, but it is certain that, in IBD, the balance of the gut microbiome is disturbed.

No Microbiome, No IBD

Studies with rodents show that the microbiome is decisive for the development of IBD. Sterile reared mice with a genetic tendency to intestinal inflammation only become ill when they were transferred a gut flora (Sellon et al. 1998). In humans, too, under certain circumstances, the course of the disease can be improved by decimating the gut flora with antibiotics. Sometimes, surgical shutdown of intestinal sections, which are then bacteria-free, can cause the inflammation to subside. In IBD patients, the diversity of bacteria is reduced, and certain species typical for the gut flora of healthy individuals are underrepresented. In the typical microbiome of IBD patients, anti-inflammatory bacterial species are reduced (Machiels et al. 2014). During disease flare-ups, the pattern of the bacterial community is different than in quiet phases (Halfvarson et al. 2017). Thus, the microbiome has a decisive influence on the disease process, but other environmental influences also determine who gets sick or stays healthy; these especially include smoking and diet (Rizello et al. 2019).

However, a multitude of inherited genes, by count, over 200, also contribute more or less strongly to the disease risk. Many of the risk genes for IBD are involved in the constant remodeling of the intestine. The approximately 32 square meters of our intestinal mucosa are one of the most active tissues of the body and are completely replaced every 3–4 days "while in operation". In order for functions such as digestion and immune defense not to suffer, the processes of cell growth, cell exchange, and repair are precisely coordinated. Even the smallest errors in these processes can lead to major disturbances, which may then make the intestinal barrier permeable. Other risk genes cause a thinner mucus layer in the affected individuals, so that intestinal bacteria can more easily come into contact with the cells of the intestinal epithelium (Degenhard and Franke 2017). Especially in the case of injuries, infections, or other disturbances, this can lead to inflammation.

A good example of the role of inherited genes is provided by the sensor protein NOD2: When it recognizes certain components of the bacterial cell wall, it triggers cells of the intestinal epithelium, known as Paneth cells, for the production of antibacterial agents. These molecules are then released into the mucus layer of the intestinal surface and keep bacteria at bay. In individuals whose NOD2 gene is crippled due to mutations, this process does not work. Bacteria that feed on mucus then migrate into the mucus layer and damage it. This makes the intestinal barrier permeable, and the immune system comes into contact with bacterial components and reacts with inflammation (Fukui 2016).

The Unwanted World Record of the Faroe Islands

Scandinavian countries are usually at the top when it comes to listing the prevalence of IBD and other inflammatory diseases. In a Europe-wide epidemiological study, it was noticed that the Faroe Islands, an archipelago in the North Atlantic, halfway between Norway and Iceland, are the absolute leaders, having the highest number of new IBD cases worldwide, namely, about 82 per 100,000 inhabitants annually (Burisch et al. 2014). This value is about 20 times higher than in European countries with a low IBD rate and twice as high as in other Scandinavian countries. Interestingly, these high values did not exist in the past, because, in the 1960s, when the Faroe Islands were still poor fishing islands, IBD was very rare. Only in the most recent decades, when prosperity came through salmon farming and fishing, did the number of new cases also increase in this remote corner of the world to ten times the initial value (Hammer et al. 2016).

A place with such a high IBD rate should be ideally suited for tracing the causes of IBD. What peculiarities are there? What genetic background do the people have? How do they eat, where do they live, what do they work at, what do they do in their free time? In response to my inquiry, Turid Hammer, the first author of the Faroe study, told me that the causes are not yet known, but many investigations are underway. And: I am cordially invited to see for myself. A visit in the summer would be best, because the other seasons are quite uncomfortable, with storm, fog and sub-zero temperatures. We arranged to meet at the end of May and I flew via Copenhagen to Tórshavn, the "smallest capital in the world", as the advertisement says.

The first inhabitants of the islands were outlaws from the Scandinavian mainland, who got their wives in Ireland and England, as I learned later. Since then, the population has steadily grown over the centuries, but only a few immigrants from outside have been added. As Pal Weihe, chief physician of the health center and professor of occupational medicine and public health explained, there are, therefore, several hereditary diseases on the Faroe Islands that are very rare elsewhere. However, IBD is not one of them; otherwise, the disease would have appeared earlier. The Faroese have the highest number of smokers compared to other Nordic countries, but the values are not so high that they would explain the higher IBD risk. Excessive use of medications, which could have an influence on IBD risk, is not in evidence. Likewise, epidemiological studies showed no influence of pollutants to which humans are exposed through the consumption of fish and other marine animals (Hammer et al. 2019).

What else could explain the high IBD rate on the Faroe Islands? The inhabitants, even the islands are far away in the Atlantic, have the same standard of living as other Scandinavian countries. Could peculiarities in diet be the cause? The stores carry the usual range of foods. Also, fruit and vegetables are available in good selection, albeit at elevated prices. According to the nutrition specialist Anna Sofia Veyhe from the hospital in Tórshavn, the eating habits on the Faroe Islands in recent decades have changed just as they have elsewhere in Scandinavia. People consume more highly processed foods, such as frozen pizza, ready-to-eat meals and sweets, and the consumption of sugary drinks has greatly increased. No wonder, then, that obesity is on the rise, especially among children. In contrast, the diet on the Faroe Islands used to be simple, consisting of bread or porridge, potatoes, dairy products, the local vegetables kohlrabi and rutabaga, as well as (fermented) fish and sheep or whale meat. My conclusion: Certainly, the diet on the Faroe Islands was healthier in the past, but it does not deviate significantly from the Scandinavian pattern. Therefore, there is no reason to assume that diet alone is responsible for the IBD rate being twice as high.

I asked if there are any peculiarities in the lifestyle that could explain the IBD rate. The landscape on the islands is typically Scandinavian: mountainous nature, albeit without forests. In between are scattered small towns with wooden houses, often in typical rust red. Tórshavn is grouped around a harbor with a historic town center, around which a small town has grown, with modern Scandinavian houses, often single-family or terraced, mostly spotlessly clean, and with middle-class cars parked outside. In the outskirts, glass office buildings, a shopping center and branches of car companies testify to the area's prosperity. What strikes me: Not only are the streets asphalted, but many houses also have concrete yards, and even the garden paths are concreted or filled with gravel. People probably want to prevent weeds or disorder from spreading anywhere. Like elsewhere, the vast majority of the population leads a modern life, has a job involving predominantly sedentary work, shops in the supermarket and only has contact with nature on summer weekends.

How different life on the Faroe Islands used to be is shown by old photos: Instead of asphalted streets and concreted yards, there were unpaved paths with numerous puddles where children played and sheep roamed. Pets were the norm. Vegetables were grown in the home garden. Dust and dirt were part of daily life. Thus, people were constantly in contact with environmental microbes. Presumably, under these conditions, people suffered more often from infections and had worms and other parasites, so that their immune system was strongly shaped in childhood and constantly challenged later. Today, on the other hand, the cleanliness of the places, the tidiness and the concreted open spaces catch the eye. The contact with environmental microbes, which tolerate the immune system, has probably decreased drastically compared to the past, but not more than in other regions of Scandinavia.

But why is the IBD rate twice as high as on the Scandinavian mainland? One factor, also emphasized by Pal Weihe, is a possible lack of vitamin D. This key factor for the immune response is activated from a precursor when UV radiation from the sun hits the skin. In northern latitudes, UV radiation is relatively low, which could explain the higher IBD disease rates in Scandinavia. On the Faroe Islands, this effect could be even more pronounced, because here, in the rough, rainy climate of the North Atlantic, the cloud cover is denser, and the UV radiation is therefore lower than elsewhere. In addition, due to the mostly bad weather, life takes place mainly indoors. Perhaps the Faroese therefore are being deprived of the UV radiation of the sun even more than elsewhere.

But what has driven the IBD incidence so high since the 1960s? The most plausible answer to me seems to be a combination effect of unfavorable factors that come together on the Faroe Islands. In all likelihood, unhealthy diet, obesity, little exercise, lack of contact with environmental bacteria and low vitamin D levels come together to cause IBD in people who are genetically susceptible. The lack of vitamin D is now being countered by supplementing the milk, a relatively easy step to accomplish. To prevent the disease, the Faroese would probably have to turn all the screws and make their lives healthier all around, including more contact with microbes. According to the latest state of research, it would be important to start with toddlers in order to program their immune system for tolerance, and thus reduce the likelihood of inflammatory diseases later in life (Fig. 5.2).

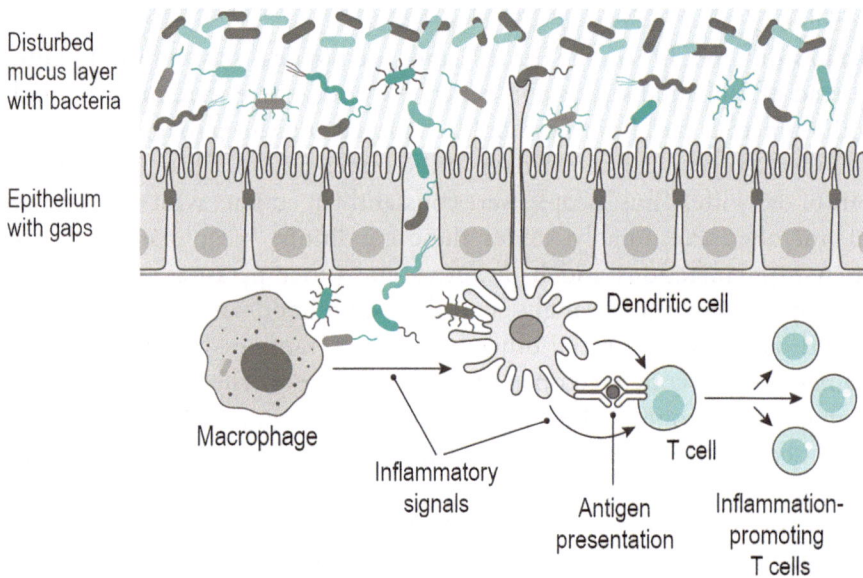

Fig. 5.2 Development of chronic inflammatory bowel diseases. When the intestinal barrier is disturbed, macrophages and dendritic cells come into contact with bacterial components and produce inflammation-promoting cytokines. Under their influence, T cells develop that initiate inflammation. (© Scorpio Verlag in Europa Verlage GmbH, München. Reproduced with permission)

Type 1 Diabetes (T1D)

The Two Forms of Diabetes

People with diabetes mellitus, also known as sugar disease in layman's terms, suffer from an excess of glucose ("grape sugar") in the blood and body fluids. While, in healthy people, the sugar level is adjusted to a physiological level by the hormone insulin, this regulation fails in diabetes. The disorder can arise in two different ways, hence the distinction between type 1 and type 2 diabetes:

Type 1 diabetes is caused by a lack of insulin. The reason for this is the destruction of insulin-producing cells of the pancreas by inflammation. T1D accounts for about 5–10% of the total number of diabetes cases and mainly occurs in children and adolescents ("juvenile diabetes").

Type 2 diabetes is caused by malfunction of the insulin receptors. The reasons for this are the decline of body functions with age ("age-related diabetes") or an overload of the receptors due to permanently high sugar concentrations in the blood ("insulin resistance"). This disorder is often associated with obesity. 90 to 95% of all diabetes cases are type 2 diabetes.

So, only T1D is an inflammatory disease, and is therefore addressed here, while type 2 diabetes is diet- or age-related. T1D is a typical civilization disease, which has always existed as a rare disease, but has increased significantly in industrialized countries in recent decades. The highest rates of T1D occur in Finland, where about 0.9% of the population is affected and about 60 new cases per 100,000 are added each year.

A Europe-wide study shows that, between 1989 and 2013, the frequency of new cases more than doubled in the 26 countries studied (Patterson et al. 2019). In contrast, the disease is still hardly known in many countries with a relatively low standard of living, such as Venezuela, Pakistan or Colombia.

Factors of the "Western lifestyle" have been discussed as the cause for the strong increase in T1D, mostly related to the microbiome. Among other things, the decline in breastfeeding of children was suspected as cause, and broad-based studies have shown that babies born by caesarean section have a doubled T1D risk (Harjutsalo et al. 2008). In T1D patients, immune tolerance is disturbed, as they develop fewer regulatory T cells, which dampen immune responses with their cytokines (Marfil-Garza et al. 2020). Genetic factors only have a relatively small share of the disease risk, at about 10% (Pociot and Lermark 2016).

The Disease T1D

The disease usually starts in childhood or adolescence. The typical sign of emerging T1D in children is a combination of pathologically increased thirst, correspondingly increased urine output and voracious appetite. The patients lose a lot of weight and often suffer from vomiting, calf cramps and abdominal pain, fatigue and weakness. Depressive moods and visual and concentration disorders are also common. The disturbed sugar metabolism poses an immediate acute danger, but also carries the risk of long-term damage.

The acute danger to T1D patients is caused by ketoacidosis, a condition that occurs when the body can no longer absorb enough glucose for its energy supply from the blood. It then switches to fat as an energy source and breaks down fat reserves. This process, however, liberates substances (for example, acetone) that lower the pH of the blood. Too precipitous a drop in this value leads to acidification of the blood, leading to symptoms of poisoning such as nausea, vomiting, abdominal pain, fatigue and changes in consciousness. Without treatment, coma and death can result.

The long-term damage caused by too high blood sugar levels comes mainly through damage to the blood vessels. Damage to large blood vessels causes a tenfold increased risk in T1D patients of cardiovascular diseases such as heart attack or stroke. Damage to small blood vessels can lead to blindness, kidney failure and nerve damage, to different degrees depending on the individual. The poor wound healing of T1D patients, especially on the legs, is due to vascular damage. It can, under certain circumstances, require amputation of feet.

The only effective therapy consists in the administration of insulin preparations that replace the body's own insulin. In this process, genetically engineered insulin proteins are used that have been specifically modified in certain stretches. These modifications cause a slower breakdown in the blood, and the molecules thus have a longer lasting effect. With these analogs, an insulin supply can be achieved that comes close to natural conditions. However, even such high-tech treatment does not cure the disease; affected people must constantly control and treat themselves, must submit to lifelong restrictions and have a shortened life expectancy overall.

Origin of the Disease

To understand the disease, one must consider the function of insulin: The ß-cells are located, together with other hormone-producing cells, in small cell islands (hence the name "insulin") in the pancreatic tissue (Fig. 5.3). One has

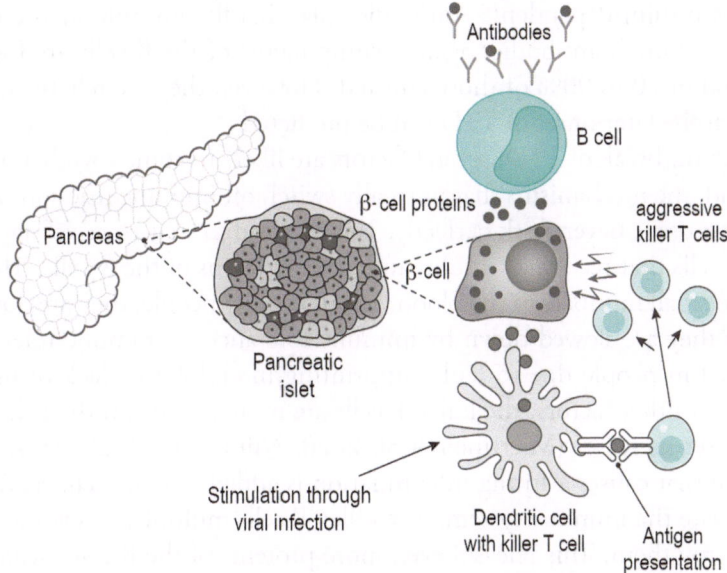

Fig. 5.3 Development of Type 1 Diabetes. Proteins of the ß-cells of the pancreas are presented by dendritic cells and activate dormant self-reactive killer T cells. This process is enhanced when the immune system is stimulated by viral infection and the offspring of the Killer T cells destroy ß-cells. B cells form antibodies against ß-cell proteins, but they do not contribute to the disease

about 1 million of these mini organs. The ß-cells constantly release small amounts of insulin, but increase their production when, for example, after a sweet meal, the concentration of glucose in the blood rises. The insulin binds to receptors on the cell surface of, for example, muscle cells, which then activate transport proteins to transport glucose into the cell interior. There, the sugar is burned for energy production. If the uptake of glucose into the cells does not work, the sugar in the blood and in other body fluids reaches high concentrations, with the previously described consequences.

In people with a genetic predisposition, certain T cells, the "killer T cells", attack the insulin-producing ß-cells and destroy them. The attack is highly specific and targets components, which only occur in the ß cells. Other killer T cells react to protein fragments of the insulin, which have been chemically altered through cell stress, and therefore are recognized as foreign by the immune system (Thomaidou et al. 2018; Kent 2017). The attack usually begins long before the disease is diagnosed, and can last for months or years. Only when a large proportion of the ß-cells are destroyed does the amount of insulin produced become insufficient. Then, the blood sugar level rises and the previously described damage to the blood vessels begins: The patient becomes insulin-dependent. Antibodies play hardly any role in the disease process, although antibodies against components of the ß-cells are found in the blood of 70 to 90% of those affected. However, they are reliable markers by which the later onset of T1D can be predicted.

For an outbreak of T1D, several factors are likely to come together: On the one hand, the mechanisms that normally switch off immune reactions against one's own tissue never work perfectly. This can lead to "self-reactive" aggressive killer T cells that recognize insulin and other proteins of the ß-cells. They circulate in small numbers in the blood, but in healthy people, they are dormant, because they are slowed down by immune tolerance. If immune tolerance is weakened in people due to faulty imprinting in childhood, lack of microbe contact, or other factors, the killer T cells are more active and the risk of diabetes onset increases (Miettinen et al. 2020; Niinistö et al. 2017). If a viral infection that causes a strong inflammation is added, the messengers released can activate the immune system. The killer T cells multiply, attack the ß-cells and destroy them. This releases even more proteins of the ß-cells, which further activates the killer T cells, stimulates inflammation and causes more cells to die. Over the course of months or years, insulin production therefore continues to decline. An infection with Coxsackie viruses, which cause respiratory diseases, has been identified as a risk factor in children in the first 3 months of life. There is also suspicion that immune responses against components of the viruses recognize and attack proteins of the ß-cells as well (Bason et al. 2013).

The Role of the Microbiome in T1D

In T1D patients, many studies have observed a reduction in bacterial diversity and a shift in balances between species in the gut, as also occurs in other inflammatory diseases. A typical pattern in T1D is a decrease in bacteria that produce short-chain fatty acids, so the inflammation brake suffers (Siljander et al. 2019).

Influences that affect the infant immune system in the first months and years of life are of great importance for the development of T1D. During this phase, in which the microbiome significantly shapes the immune system, a balanced ratio of stimuli is important. On the one hand, it is beneficial if bacteria that produce many short-chain fatty acids, and thus apply the inflammation brake, dominate in the microbiome. On the other hand, a certain degree of inflammatory stimuli is obviously necessary to train anti-inflammatory circuits. In this context, for example, the bacterial LPS presented in the microbiome chapter, a surface component of gram-negative bacteria, is important.

If one wants to check the influence of the microbiome on the risk for T1D, one must follow the intestinal flora and its influence on immune responses of children with high or low risk for T1D in detail over a long period of time. Where could such studies best be conducted? Let's remember the region of Karelia, mentioned in Chap. 2 (Section "The Iron Curtain"), in the Finnish-Russian border region. In highly developed Finland, the number of new T1D cases is about six times higher than in rural, underdeveloped Russian Karelia. This constellation has motivated an international research team to conduct a comprehensive study to investigate the connection between T1D, gut flora, and the shaping of the immune system.

The research team, led by Ramnik Xavier from the National Institute of Health in Bethesda, MD, USA, followed a cohort of 222 children in Northern Europe from birth to the age of three (further follow-up of the cohort is ongoing). 74 children with a comparable genetic risk for T1D came from the Finnish and Russian parts of Karelia, respectively. For comparison, 74 children from Estonia, a country that has developed rapidly since the collapse of the Soviet Union, were also studied. Rates of allergies and autoimmune responses there are now similar to those in Scandinavia.

Analyses of the immune response showed significant differences between Russian children on the one hand and children from Finland and Estonia on the other: Autoimmune antibodies against insulin-producing cells were found in just under 2% of Russian children, while the proportion in Finnish and Estonian children was about five times higher. Thus, it was expected that Russian children would develop far less T1D than children from Finland and Estonia (Vatanen et al. 2016).

What was the connection between these findings and the children's gut flora? The analyses showed that the gut flora of children from all three regions had a roughly equal, relatively low proportion of Escherichia coli. In Russian children, bifidobacteria and related species dominated in the early phase of childhood, but were gradually displaced by Bacteroides, which, by the end of the third year of life, constituted the vast majority of bacterial groups. In children from Finland and Estonia, on the other hand, a large proportion of the gut flora consisted of Bacteroides from the start, while bifidobacteria only made up a small proportion (Fig. 5.4). When considering how these differences could affect disease risk, researchers came across LPS: the structure of this surface molecule varies among bacterial species, and thus also has different effects on the immune system.

Experiments with mice showed that LPS from E. coli strongly stimulated the animals' immune cells upon first contact. Further contact, however, led to the cells becoming accustomed to the bacterium-specific substance and made

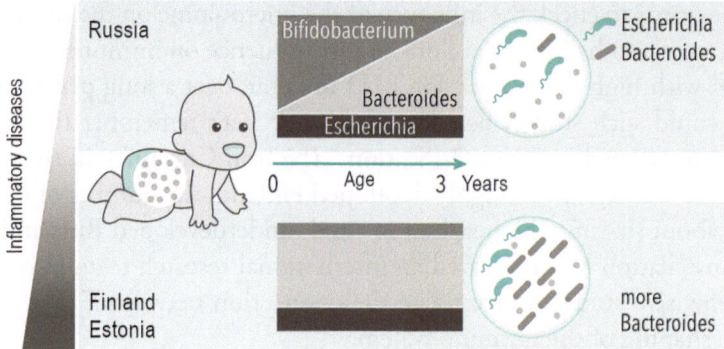

Fig. 5.4 Regional differences in the shaping of immune tolerance in the first years of life. In toddlers from Russia, who have a low risk of inflammatory diseases later in life, bifidobacteria dominate at an early age, allowing E. coli to shape immune tolerance. In children from Finland and Estonia, Bacteroides dominate from early childhood and suppress the shaping of the immune system by E. coli. (Modified after Vatanen et al. 2016. © Scorpio Verlag in Europa Verlage GmbH, München. Reproduced with permission)

them immune tolerant, as described in Chap. 4 on the microbiome (see the section "Microbial Danger Signals"). In contrast, the LPS from Bacteroides bacteria did not stimulate the immune cells of the mice, and therefore did not trigger the mechanisms of immune tolerance. On the contrary, LPS from Bacteroides even prevented stimulation of the cells by E. coli LPS when LPS from both bacteria was given in cell cultures at the same time. Through this effect, the Bacteroides LPS neutralized the tolerizing effect of E. coli LPS.

These data explain the different disease risks for the children: Since the Finnish and Estonian children were primarily exposed to Bacteroides LPS from the start, according to Ramnik Xavier, the necessary stimulation by E. coli LPS did not occur. Thus, their immune system was less strongly programmed for immune tolerance, and this increased the risk of a later T1D disease (Vatanen et al. 2016).

Multiple Sclerosis (MS)

The Disease MS

MS is one of the inflammatory diseases that appeared in earlier centuries, but apparently were rare, thus attracting attention. An example of this is the story of Saint Lidwina of Schiedam, a city near Rotterdam. According to the legend, the 15-year-old Lidwina fell while ice skating, broke a rib, and never recovered. The tradition says that she collided with a friend, but it is quite conceivable that she fell because she had vision or balance disorders. After her accident, she developed typical MS-related mobility impairments and severe pain. At the age of 19, both her legs were paralyzed, and her vision was impaired. Additional ailments followed. Until her death at the age of 53, Lidwina's condition deteriorated in phases. Even during her lifetime, she was mythically glorified and attracted crowds of people. The city administration of Schiedam promoted this rare attraction by spreading the word that Lidwina needed neither food nor sleep. After her death, her grave became a pilgrimage site and, in 1890, Lidwina, known as "the sufferer", was canonized. Today, she is simultaneously a patron saint of the sick and of ice skaters.

The saint's disease shows so many symptoms of MS that it is now considered the first description of that condition. Typical of this medical history is, among other things, the fact that a very young woman is affected. The first symptoms of MS occur in most patients between the ages of 15 and 40. They are caused by inflammations that damage the brain, optic nerves, and spinal cord. Initially, isolated failures occur, such as visual, balance, or sensory disorders, which completely disappear, but then reappear after several weeks, months, or even years. With the repeated disease relapses, which last several days or weeks, further disabilities such as paralysis are added. In the further course, the symptoms no longer recede between the episodes of the disease, so that the state of health permanently deteriorates. The likelihood of relapses is increased by infections, such as flu or viral intestinal diseases. However, there are also forms of MS that run continuously without pronounced episodes from the beginning.

Often, the first symptoms noticed are visual disturbances caused by inflammation in the area of the optic nerve or the processing brain areas. If certain nerve pathways are affected by the inflammations, numbness, pain, and cramps can occur in the hands or legs, for example; inflammations in the cerebellum or brainstem can cause swallowing disorders, speech disorders, or impaired movement coordination. Also, choppy speech, trembling movements, or spastic paralysis can occur. Body functions that are involuntarily controlled, such as reflexes, digestion and excretion, or sexual activities, can be impaired or fail. Also typical is the total lack of energy in patients, referred to as "fatigue"; emotional outbursts and cognitive disorders can also occur. In the late stage of the disease, dementia can also occur. The diversity of MS complicates diagnosis.

Spread and Increase of MS

As with other inflammation-related diseases, an increase in MS has been observed in industrialized countries over the past decades. A good example is provided by figures from Denmark, where data has been collected in a national MS register since 1956. In Denmark in 1950, 0.059% of the population had MS, while the frequency had risen to almost five times that value by 2020 (MS International Federation 2020). As in other countries, MS has particularly increased among women. In Europe, Germany, Austria, and the Scandinavian countries are among the top group, while MS is less common in the Mediterranean region (Kingwell et al. 2013).

The increase in MS is associated with modern lifestyles in developed countries. American studies, in which the MS rates of US citizens of African and European descent were examined, support this view. Here, it was shown that lifestyle, and not ethnic affiliation, determines the MS risk. Essential decisions that affect the MS risk take place in childhood or early adolescence. Anyone who grew up in an area with a low MS risk, and only immigrated to an area with a high risk as an adult, retains the low disease risk programmed in childhood. On the other hand, if you immigrate as a child to a high-risk area, you will later develop the usual high disease risk found there (Koch-Henriksen and Soerensen 2010).

An important factor that co-determines the frequency of MS is contact with microbes. Infections play a role here, because individuals who are infected with the stomach bacterium Helicobacter pylori, with parasitic worms or the parasite Toxoplasma gondii, have a lower risk of developing MS (Wendel-Haga and Celius 2017). The gut flora also has an influence, because, in people with MS, inflammation-promoting bacterial species are more prevalent than in healthy people, while inflammation-inhibiting bacteria, which dampen the immune response by producing short-chain fatty acids, are underrepresented (Chen et al. 2016a, b; Jangi et al. 2016). However, in this case too, it is not clear whether the disturbed balance of the bacterial flora is the cause or consequence of the disease. The fact that the disease can be triggered or worsened by transferring the gut bacteria from MS patients to mice argues for their role as a trigger (Berer et al. 2017; Cekanaviciute et al. 2017).

The Massacre in the Brain

In MS, the immune system causes a veritable massacre among the nerve cells of the brain, spinal cord, and optic nerves through inflammation. The main target is the myelin sheath of the nerve fibers. To understand the underlying processes, one should have the scene of the event in mind: The human brain consists of about 170 billion cells, of which about 50% are nerve cells (neurons) and the other 50% glial cells, which support the neurons in their functions.

Typical neurons consist of a cell body, several highly branched extensions, the dendrites, and a nerve fiber, the axon. The dendrites make contact with the dendrites of other nerve cells with their relatively short extensions, and are thus responsible for the interconnection of the nerve cells. The axons, on the other hand, are responsible for conducting the electrical nerve signals over longer distances. They can be up to one meter long and connect the nerve cell from which they originate with another nerve cell, a muscle or a gland cell. For the electrical stimulus conduction over longer distances to work, axons are surrounded by an insulating layer, the myelin sheath, like an electrical cable is surrounded by a plastic sheath.

The myelin sheath is formed by certain glial cells, the oligodendrocytes. Their most important protein is myelin. Each of these cells wraps a section of the axon in several layers. One can vividly imagine a neuron with its insulating myelin sheath by thinking of a bandage wrapped in several layers around a wounded finger. In MS, T cells recognize the myelin protein of the myelin sheath of axons and trigger inflammations.

The tumult attracts further inflammatory cells and activates them, so that the focus expands and a witch's cauldron is created in which the immune response indiscriminately destroys tissue. In addition, a further wave of cells now migrates from blood vessels into the inflammation focus, including many phagocytes, whose task is to clear away the destroyed tissue. After some time, such local Inflammation foci come to a halt again, although it is not clear what causes the calming. As a result, dead, scarred areas remain in the brain tissue and corresponding functional failures result (Filippi et al. 2018).

The typical, relapsing course of inflammation in MS patients comes about through a repetition of the previously described processes: T cells are repeatedly activated in the body by an unknown trigger, migrate into the brain and initiate an almost autonomously running inflammation there. In later stages of the disease, inflammatory cells are usually not only found in local foci, but also scattered throughout the tissue of the brain and spinal cord. The nerve tissue destroyed by inflammation can only be regenerated to a limited extent, and so the damage accumulates: More and more neurons lose their conductivity or die off, so that signal transmission is extremely slowed down and eventually fails. This leads to the previously described failures of sensory perception, movement and involuntarily controlled body functions. In addition to direct destruction, the cytokines released also cause constant fatigue and exhaustion.

There are numerous modern treatment methods, including the use of genetically engineered interferon-ß and various monoclonal antibodies. They reduce the symptoms, delay new relapses and slow down the progression of the disease. However, current therapies cannot prevent the health of those affected from deteriorating in the long term and the permanent restrictions from increasing; even today, people with MS have a lower life expectancy (Filippi et al. 2018).

Immunological Cross-reactions as Triggers of MS?

MS is due to an interaction of genetic factors and environmental factors, which together lead to inflammatory responses irreversibly damaging the central nervous system. Over 200 risk genes are known, which collectively determine the probability of the disease occurring to about 30%. Most of these genes have an influence on the expression of immune responses. The HLA-DRB1*15:01 protein, whose function is to present protein fragments to T cells, and thus stimulate them to activate and divide, has the most significant influence (Hollenbach and Oksenberg 2015). People with this gene variant have a significantly increased risk of MS. Other important risk genes enhance the formation of inflammation-promoting cytokines. However, environmental factors have a greater influence than genetic factors. In addition to smoking, low vitamin D levels and childhood obesity, adolescent infections with the Epstein-Barr virus (EBV) pose a significant risk (Dobson and Giovannoni 2019).

Why does EBV fit the pattern of a pathogen that triggers MS? To explain this, one has to go a bit further. EBV belongs to the family of herpes viruses, which have in common a usually somewhat peaceful long-term relationship with their host. Everyone knows the herpes simplex virus, which slumbers in the trigeminal nerve of the face and causes the well-known lip blisters in case of stress, too much UV light or after infections. EBV has a similar biology. More than 95% of the average population has gone through this infection, as can be demonstrated in antibody tests. The transmission takes place with saliva and through droplet or smear infection, usually in early childhood. In toddlers, the infection is inconspicuous and protects against later disease caused by the virus.

However, if one does not get infected as a toddler, but only later, the virus causes mononucleosis, also known as Pfeiffer's glandular fever, a febrile disease with swelling of Lymph nodes and strong proliferation of B cells. Since mononucleosis mainly occurs in adolescents and can be transmitted through kissing, it is also referred to as the kissing disease or student fever. As a rule, the infection heals on its own.

However, the virus does not completely disappear: After healing, it lies inactive in the B cells and is kept in check by the immune system. Under stress or after infections, the pressure of the immune response decreases. Then, the virus can become active again, primarily producing viruses in the salivary glands that can be transmitted. This temporary reactivation of EBV, which strongly stimulates the immune system each time, could explain the disease relapses in MS.

In particular, the theory would fit if there were dormant immune responses against myelin protein that are awakened during the reactivation of the virus by inflammatory signals. In search of such immune responses, researchers isolated T cells from the brains of people with MS and tested which proteins the cells recognize. They came across the enzyme fucose synthase, which is involved in sugar metabolism in several types of gut bacteria. The structures of the bacterial enzyme show structural similarity in certain sections with a fragment of the myelin protein. T cells of MS patients, which recognized the bacterial protein, also reacted simultaneously to the human myelin protein (Planas et al. 2018). Such "cross-reacting" T cells could attack the myelin sheath when they are activated by infections or the braking mechanisms of immune tolerance are disturbed.

Molecular cross-reactions can also explain the cause of other diseases, as shown in the examples of psoriasis, rheumatoid arthritis, and celiac disease in the following sections of this chapter. It must be assumed that all people have many cross-reacting T cells (and also B cells), because, on the one hand, the immune system always comes into contact with the microbes of the gut and other compartments, so that microbe-reactive immune cells are formed, while, on the other hand, there are many molecular similarities between microbes and higher animals such as humans, so that some of the microbe-reactive cells also recognize human proteins at the same time. These "self-reactive" cells usually lie dormant and are kept inactive by mechanisms of immune tolerance. However, they can be activated and multiply massively when stimulated by inflammatory processes. According to this scenario, molecular similarities between the microbiome and human proteins pose no danger in a balanced immune system. However, the situation can get out of control if the balance of immune responses is disturbed in people with an unfavorable combination of risk genes by factors such as imprinting in childhood, smoking, or an inflammation-promoting microbiome (Fig. 5.5).

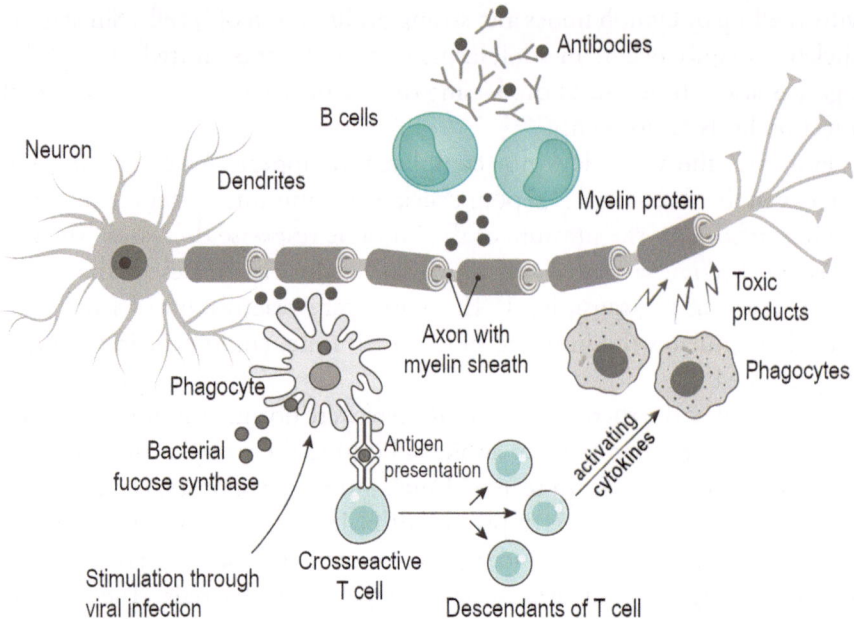

Fig. 5.5 Development of Multiple Sclerosis. Dormant self-reactive T cells, which recognize both the myelin protein of axons and bacterial fucose synthase ("cross-reaction"), are activated by inflammatory stimuli. They stimulate phagocytes to attack the myelin sheath. Antibodies against myelin protein are also formed, but they are not relevant to the disease. (© Scorpio Verlag in Europa Verlage GmbH, München. Reproduced with permission)

Psoriasis

The Disease Psoriasis

In psoriasis, skin, nails or joints are affected by inflammation, but the disease also has effects on the entire body. Psoriasis occurs in very different forms. The most common is psoriasis vulgaris: Here, sharply defined, raised and reddened areas of skin form foci ("plaques") of silvery-white scales, which usually itch severely. Often, knees, elbows and areas of the body that are mechanically stressed, as well as the scalp, are affected. The plaques can occur in isolation, but can also spread over larger areas or, in rare cases, cover the skin of the entire body. Brittle spots can form on nails ("pitted nail", "oil spot", "crumb nail"). Often, the disease occurs in weekly or monthly bouts, which completely subside in between. Other important manifestations are psoriatic arthritis, which affects the joints and their associated ligaments, and psoriasis pustulosa, in which fluid-filled blisters form at the inflamed skin sites. Psoriasis can pave the way for several other diseases, including cardiovascular diseases, type 2 diabetes, chronic inflammatory bowel diseases, and psychiatric complications.

Psoriasis is a relatively common disease, affecting more than 100 million people worldwide, predominantly in highly developed countries and particularly among people of Northern European origin. It is rare in infants, but the chances of developing it increase into adulthood. In the Western world, on average, about 2–3% of the population suffer from psoriasis. Norway, with a prevalence of 14%, is one of the most affected countries, while, for example, in Tanzania, only 0.09% of the population suffer from psoriasis (Gibbs 1996). Due to the diversity of psoriasis and the variability of diagnostic methods, it is difficult to track incidence and prevalence. A doubling of the number of cases over recent decades has been reported from very different countries, such as China, Norway and the USA. This pattern corresponds to that of other inflammatory diseases, suggesting an increased tendency towards inflammation due to the Western lifestyle.

In the development of the disease, genetic factors are decisive, but environmental factors modify the risk (Kunz et al. 2019). The probability of an identical twin becoming ill if the other twin has psoriasis is as high 65–72%. About 50 risk genes are known whose interplay determines the form and course of the disease. The most important role is played by several genes of the HLA system, with which phagocytes present protein fragments to the T cells of the immune system. In addition, in people with a predisposition for psoriasis, genes are also altered that code for cytokines and other proteins that regulate immune responses. In addition to genetic factors, factors such as smoking, obesity and sunburn significantly contribute to the risk. Apparently, in psoriasis, the balance of immune responses is particularly unstable, and so the disease process is sometimes influenced by minor disturbances, such as changes in location or diet. The inflammations flare up particularly when the balance of the immune system is upset by highly stressful events, such as after a severe flu infection, an operation, or the death of a relative.

The Interplay of Triggers

At the beginning of a psoriasis episode, there is often an irritation of the skin due to mechanical stress, sunburn or other stress. These processes activate defense and repair mechanisms in the skin cells. In the process, specific proteins are formed that, among other things, attack bacteria and activate the immune response. One protein that plays an important role in the psoriatic inflammation of many patients is the cathelicidin LL-37. This small molecule is very reactive and hooks into the surface of bacteria to destroy them. This wards off invading germs. In addition, cathelicidin supports the process of wound healing by stimulating cells to divide, and thus normally plays a positive role. However, the protein has the dangerous property of binding to DNA that is released from damaged cells. The molecule complexes resulting from cathelicidin and DNA can be recognized by cells of the innate immune response and activate them. These immune cells then attract further immune cells through cytokines and stimulate them, resulting in inflammation (Benhadou et al. 2019; Greb et al. 2016). Thus, cathelicidin also has a dark side, as it can enhance the tendency towards inflammation.

Another important element in the disease process are "self-reactive" T cells, which are constantly produced due to molecular cross-reactions with bacterial proteins, as described in the section on Multiple Sclerosis in this chapter. In healthy individuals, these cells lie dormant, but can be activated by inflammatory signals. Such signals can occur, for example, after a sunburn through cathelicidin-DNA complexes, but also through other causes. In people with psoriasis, among other things, self-reactive T cells occur against keratin 17, a protein found in the epidermis, but also in smaller amounts in many other tissues. These T cells cross-react with the M-protein of streptococci (Yunusbaeva et al. 2018). It is therefore obvious that contact with streptococci in individuals with corresponding genetic predispositions leads to the formation of T cells that also recognize keratin 17. When activated by inflammation, the self-reactive T cells attack their target protein, multiply, and further fuel the inflammation with their cytokines. These processes damage the tissue of the subcutaneous layer, but, at the same time, stimulate the keratin-forming cells of the epidermis to divide. These cells form the multilayered top layer of the skin, which is constantly renewed from below. Irritated by the inflammatory processes, the keratinocytes multiply much faster than they would in healthy skin.

In addition to activation by self-reactive T cells, however, other inflammatory stimuli also have an effect. In response, new layers of the epidermis are constantly formed and shed. The cells cannot mature and stick together. This results in the silvery, wax-like skin flakes typical of psoriasis.

However, the inflammatory processes are not limited to the skin, as keratin 17 and other target proteins of self-reactive T cells are also present in small amounts in other organs. Therefore, the disease can also spread there. This effect is referred to as "psoriatic march" and leads to psoriatic arthritis in about 40% of patients. This results in inflammation of the joints, similar to rheumatoid arthritis. In addition to many other effects, the walls of the blood vessels

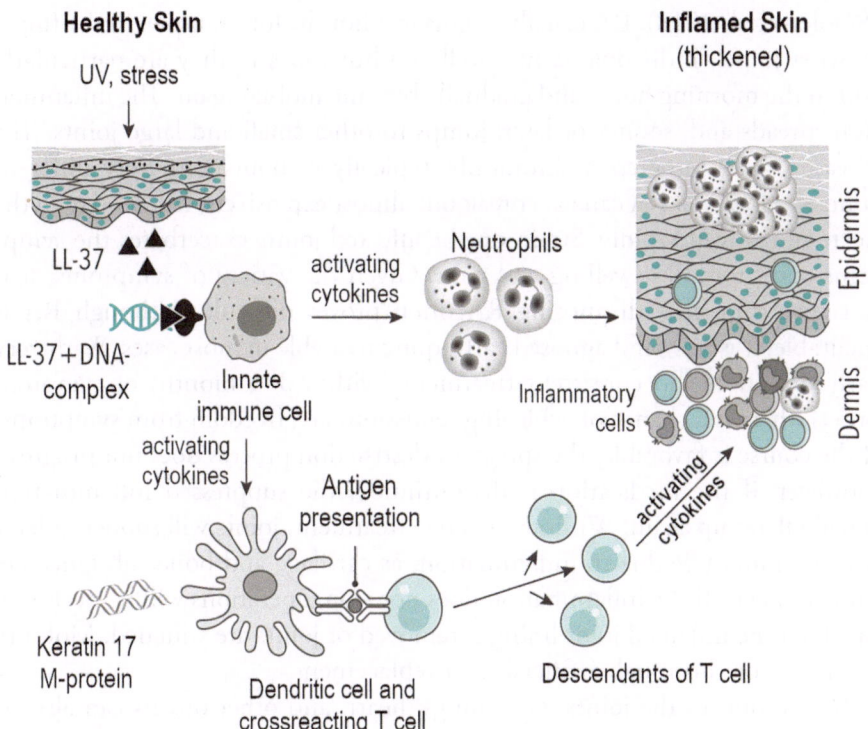

Fig. 5.6 Development of psoriasis. Left: healthy skin. Right: inflamed skin. On the one hand, after UV or other stress, the cathelicidin LL-37 is formed and binds to DNA. This complex stimulates cells of the innate immune response to produce inflammation-promoting cytokines. On the other hand, this activates dormant self-reactive T cells that recognize both keratin 17 and M-protein from streptococci ("cross-reaction"). The offspring of these T cells intensify the inflammation with their cytokines. The keratinocytes of the inflamed skin divide too quickly, so the architecture of the skin suffers. (© Scorpio Verlag in Europa Verlage GmbH, München. Reproduced with permission)

can also be damaged, which promotes high blood pressure and heart disease, making psoriasis a systemic disease (Fig. 5.6).

Rheumatoid Arthritis (RA)

The Disease RA

In everyday language, the term "rheumatism" is used for a whole group of over 100 different diseases. The most common is "Rheumatoid Arthritis" (RA), which affects approximately 0.5–1% of the population worldwide

(Smolen et al. 2018). RA usually begins insidiously, for example, in the finger or wrist joints. Individual joints swell and hurt. Often, they are particularly stiff in the morning hours and gradually become mobile again. The inflammation spreads and, sooner or later, jumps to other small and large joints. The disease usually progresses chronically, typically in bouts with very different courses. However, RA can also break out almost explosively, from 1 day to the next, and spread rapidly. Strain on the affected joints exacerbates the symptoms and promotes swelling and pain. Given the variety of symptoms, it is not surprising that diagnosing RA often proves difficult. Although RA is incurable, it is now, if diagnosed early, quite treatable in most cases. With very early detection and consistent treatment (within 3–4 months of symptom onset), there is a chance of achieving remission, i.e., freedom from symptoms. If the course is favorable, the spread or destruction process does not progress. However, if the medication is discontinued, the suppressed inflammation usually flares up again. Without effective treatment, joints will sooner or later become immobile due to inflammation, as cartilage and bone substance are broken down. If the inflammation does not stop, operations will be necessary in which the inflamed joint lining is removed or joints are stiffened. Mobility can be restored through artificial joint replacement.

In addition to the joints, eyes, lungs, heart, and other organs can also be affected, so without adequate treatment, the survival time of RA patients is significantly shortened (Smolen et al. 2018). Last but not least, patients suffer from chronic fatigue and lethargy, which is also typical of other inflammatory diseases. The saying "Rheumatism doesn't kill, but it takes life!" aptly describes this condition.

RA is one of the few inflammatory diseases whose prevalence has not increased in recent decades, so RA is not a typical civilization disease. This peculiarity is probably due to the fact that the risk of disease is about 60% determined by genetic factors. The disease can begin at any age, but RA symptoms usually occur between the ages of 40 and 70. Women are about two to three times more likely to be affected than men.

Genes that determine which protein fragments are well presented to the T cells of the immune system play a major role in the risk of disease. Individuals with certain HLA-DRB1 type genes have the highest risk for RA, but about 100 other genes are also involved in the manifestation of the disease. If genetic predisposition is combined with other risk factors, the probability of disease increases significantly. For example, smokers get sick on average about twice as often as non-smokers. However, if smokers carry one of the important HLA-DRB1 genes, their probability of developing RA is 20 times higher compared to non-smokers without a risk gene (Kallberg et al. 2011), and their disease is far less responsive to treatment than it is in non-smokers. Overweight individuals also have an increased risk of developing RA, probably due to the inflammation-promoting cytokines released by visceral fat tissue.

It is still unclear why RA occurs less frequently in some regions, such as the Mediterranean area. This protective effect could be due to the stronger sunlight in the south, which leads to the formation of more vitamin D. Other studies consider the Mediterranean diet—with its many fibers and unsaturated fatty acids—as the cause for the protective effect. However, other factors may also be responsible for the differences in frequency. For example, rheumatologists take their patients' sensitivity to "the weather" very seriously, as a worsening of symptoms in damp, cold weather is often reported, but cannot be scientifically explained. British researchers approached this question with the "Citizen Science" approach, setting up the website www.cloudywitha-chanceofpain.com, that alludes to the prognosis of the weather report "cloudy with a chance of rain". Interested parties could enter their current condition using an app on their smartphone. The smartphone simultaneously transmitted the geographical coordinates, so that the weather at the corresponding location could be called up at the same time. The data showed that, when in damp, cold weather, the sensation of pain is actually about 20% stronger than in warm, dry summer weather (Dixon 2019). No wonder then that, in earlier times, rheumatics sought out the sunny Côte d'Azur or Egypt to give their joints a sun break.

Sudden Rheumatism: A Patient Tells Her Story

For me, "rheumatism" was always a disease of old people, who have crippled hands with knotty, inflammation-deformed joints and bent, stiff fingers. Never in my life would I have thought that people who are active in life could fall ill with it, let alone me. Now, I have had Rheumatoid Arthritis (RA), the most common of the many diseases that belong to the "rheumatoid spectrum", for 5 years.

For many patients, RA begins insidiously, but for me, it set in suddenly, precisely on my 60th birthday. Initially, I had swelling and pain in my left hand, so that I could hardly move my fingers within a few hours. The family doctor suspected an allergy and prescribed an antihistamine, but by the evening, my right hand began to swell and I had excruciating pain. Both hands were then heavily bandaged, splinted and immobilized; nothing more could be done. I couldn't use either hand for the time being, and so I sat on our couch all weekend, handicapped in the truest sense of the word, with severe pain, waiting for "it" to go away. After 3–4 days, the swelling subsided, I was happy about the newly gained strength, from which I let our garden benefit. But not much came of it, because the same game started all over again: In no time, both hands were swollen and the fingers became immobile, while I suffered from excruciating pain. But now, "it" had also spread to the wrists, first one, then the other. Two days later, "it" was also in my feet!

As there was no sign of improvement—rather, the disease progressed rapidly and I continued to have very severe pain—I went to the clinic for rheumatism of a large hospital. A hallmark of rheumatism diagnosis is the so-called morning stiffness of the affected joints, especially the hands. But I didn't have this, and there were also no "rheumatism factors" (RA-typical antibodies) detectable in my blood. So, RA was ruled out as the cause of the painful swellings. The advice was to wait and see; perhaps the complaints would go away on their own. Since no diagnosis was in sight, my family doctor then tried pain therapy, giving me a strong cortisone injection with painkiller. This brought temporary relief. I was so happy that the horror was over, but, very quickly, I learned otherwise.

From this point on, our sofa in the living room was to be my bed, my apartment and my home for five long months, as I was increasingly unable to move. Five very long months, at the end of which I finally sat in a wheelchair, partly unable to walk, unable to take care of myself. Combing my hair or even cutting my fingernails—unthinkable! Opening a bottle of sparkling water to drink—forget it! Holding my cup or glass—no way! Sometimes I woke up at night in pain and then suddenly found that I couldn't get up, couldn't straighten up or even move my legs—oh God, how am I going to get to the toilet?

My functional limitations were so overwhelming that I went from zero to a hundred disabled. The crazy thing about rheumatic joints is that they lock up and simply do not move, even if you are willing to endure great pain. They just don't work at all anymore. Once, I sat on a chair in our kitchen and couldn't get up, was immobile, virtually tied down, until my husband came home from work about an hour and a half later and lifted me up and to the sofa. I had to be pushed in the wheelchair, because I could not move the wheels with my hands myself. The slightest strain on my hands immediately triggered new swelling and pain. Once, my husband had gone to work in the morning and had accidentally left no food for me on the sofa—but I could not go to the kitchen alone to get something from the fridge. I couldn't call someone and ask for help either, because I couldn't hold the phone. Luckily, a neighbor happened to visit and took care of me. And the fatigue—in the end, I was just hanging out on my sofa, feeling nothing but tired, tired, tired ... like having a permanent flu, but without a virus. I could neither make phone calls nor type—working on the computer or writing emails were not my thing for a long time. When someone came to visit, I fell asleep after about 45 minutes.

During this time, I went through a whole odyssey, from the emergency doctor, whom we had to call when I suddenly couldn't move my leg anymore, to the family doctor, an allergist, and rheumatologist. Since I had no morning stiffness and no RA-typical antibodies in my blood, I still could not get a diagnosis. Only when my cardiologist, whom I visited in a wheelchair, suspected rheumatism did things started to roll.

The start of therapy thus began about 5 months after the onset of the disease. I was prescribed cortisone and methotrexate (a drug that inhibits cell division). Of course, this did not immediately end the disease, as I had to learn, and, what's more, the symptoms initially worsened. Also, the weekly dose of methotrexate was very unpleasant and incapacitated me for a whole day. In the first weeks, I rolled into the doctor's office in a wheelchair. A little later, I could walk a bit again, but the paths in the clinic and from the doctor's office to the diagnosis made me break out in sweat. Only when I changed doctors did I finally get a biologic, a monoclonal antibody against the cytokine TNF-α, which neutralizes this messenger substance. Over the months and years, the joints normalized again and the grueling pain, the weakness and the fatigue disappeared.

Five years later, I am grateful that modern medications permit me a somewhat normal life. However, this is only possible with my weekly injection of a TNF blocker. As soon as I tried to extend the periods between injections, the rheumatism came back. Several times, I had to change the medication, because it lost its effectiveness. For a while, I was able to stop taking the methotrexate, but now, I have to take it again to prevent the formation of antibodies against the biologic. I have to take very good care of myself, because as soon as I overexert myself, my hands swell up again and my knees cause problems. Longer walks are not possible, and all walking and gardening must be carefully limited in their doses. I am easily fatigued and can no longer tolerate many foods that I used to enjoy. I have to completely avoid dairy products and can only tolerate home-cooked food. Are these the effects of methotrexate? It is hard to be sure, as I hear from acquaintances that they tolerate the medication well.

I think that the tenacious belief that I can be healed has helped me a lot. I did not resign myself to a fate as a rheumatism patient, e.g., remodeling the bathroom to be barrier-free, but rather I informed myself about treatment methods and aids and asked the doctors probing questions. Stays in southern

France, where we spent two winters with friends, also helped me. However, it is not clear to me how a single person can cope with such a disease, because support is enormously important. So, warning to all singles: Make sure you have a partner before you get something like this (haha!).

Why Do the Joints Become Inflamed?

To understand RA, it is helpful to imagine the main scene of the action, the joint gap. Let's take, as an example, the finger joint. A finger joint, this movable connection between two finger bones, is surrounded by a joint capsule made of dense connective tissue. The two finger bones protrude into the fluid-filled capsule as the joint head and the joint socket. In between lies the joint space. The bones are covered with cartilage, which acts as a shock absorber. In addition, the gelatinous joint fluid also absorbs shocks and lubricates the colliding cartilage surfaces. The joint capsule is lined with a thin inner skin, the synovium. This inner skin is well vascularized; its blood vessels supply the joint with nutrients and transport waste products away.

In most patients, the disease has already developed a long time before the typical joint inflammations become noticeable. In this symptom-free early stage, certain antibodies can already be detected in many patients that are crucially involved in the disease, even if further events then lead to the outbreak. There are antibodies that bind to other antibodies and are referred to as "rheumatoid factors". They glue these antibodies together, so to speak, and form large complexes, the "immune complexes", which attach to the walls of blood vessels. Immune cells can recognize these immune complexes with their receptors. As a result, they are activated, release aggressive substances and attract other immune cells with cytokines. The resulting inflammation damages the walls of the blood vessels and makes them permeable. Then, fluid enters the joint space and the surrounding tissue, causing swelling to develop (Fig. 5.7).

Beyond these inflammatory processes, antibodies against certain proteins that contain the rare amino acid citrulline are important. Such proteins naturally occur in the joint space, but through cell stress, such as smoking, normal proteins in the body also change, and can then contain citrulline. Also, enzymes of the bacterium Porphyromonas gingivalis, which lives in the pockets of inflamed teeth, citrullinate proteins of the host, and thus change their structure. These altered proteins are recognized by the immune system of individuals with certain subtypes of the immune response gene HLA DRB1. Then, especially in patients with severe disease progression, ACPA (anti

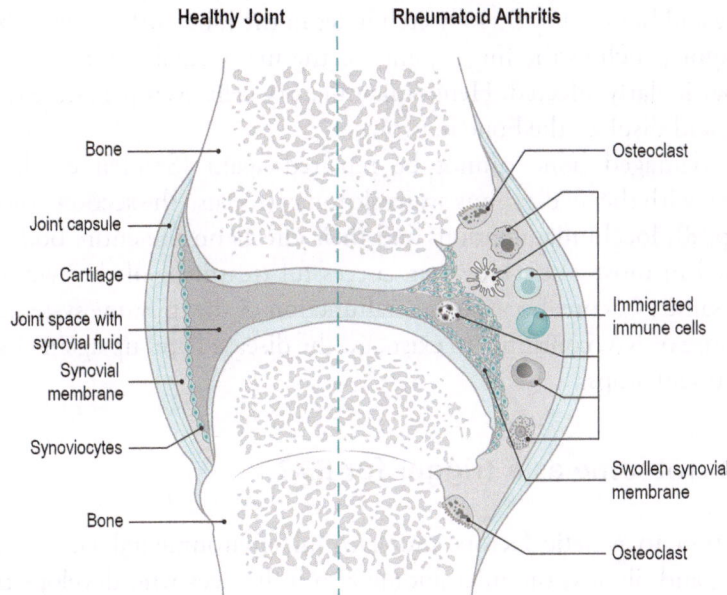

Fig. 5.7 Diagram of a joint in Rheumatoid Arthritis. In the attacked joint (right), immune cells have migrated into the joint space. With their signals, they initiate a proliferation of the joint lining and attack the cartilage. Activated osteoclasts destroy the bone. (Modified after Smolen et al. 2018. © Scorpio Verlag in Europa Verlage GmbH, München. Reproduced with permission)

citrullinated protein antibodies) are formed. These antibodies pass through the damaged blood vessels into the joint space and bind there to the citrullinated proteins. These bound antibodies are recognized by immune cells, so an inflammation is initiated. In this process, the cells of the joint lining also multiply and produce their own inflammatory messengers, which attract and activate further cells. The proliferating joint lining grows into the joint space and narrows it (Smolen et al. 2018). From the inflamed joints, however, cells also migrate out and are carried with the blood to other joints, where they start new inflammations (Lefevre et al. 2009).

The inflammatory cells in the joint space produce aggressive substances that damage the tissue and the cartilage. This narrows the joint space, which increases the friction of the bones against each other, causing the joints to be very painful and severely swollen. It is often only at this stage that the diagnosis is made. The bones themselves are also attacked. The culprits here are osteoclasts, cells that actually have an important function in the remodeling of bone substance and are equipped with particularly aggressive enzymes. The Inflammatory cytokines in the joint activate them, and their enzymes dissolve cartilage and bone. They literally etch holes in the joint surface, with the most active joints, such as the finger joints or the many small joints of the wrist, being particularly affected. Here, inflammatory cells even penetrate the bone interior and displace the bone marrow.

Such damaged bone cannot be repaired again (Smolen et al. 2018). However, with the medications available today (see also the section "Biologics" in Chap. 8), local inflammations and their effects on the entire body can be contained in most cases. However, successful treatment of the symptoms is not the same as a cure, because the malfunction of the immune system, which is the cause of RA, continues to exist and the disease flares up again as soon as the treatment stops.

The Microbiome as a Trigger for RA?

In addition to genetic factors and harmful environmental factors such as smoking and obesity, the microbiome also influences who develops the disease and how it progresses. RA patients have a reduced diversity of gut bacteria and certain, otherwise rare bacteria are overrepresented (Chen et al. 2016a, b). Perhaps what happens in the gut is even the trigger for the onset of the disease. A disease similar to RA illustrates how the onset of RA could occur.

It is noticeable that, sometimes, very specific infections of the intestine, which are accompanied by severe diarrhea, trigger a temporary, massive joint inflammation, the "reactive arthritis". Thus, individuals after an infection with, for example, the bacteria Shigella or Salmonella, or with the single-celled parasite Giardia, can get a severe inflammation of several joints, which partly forces them into a wheelchair. Usually, large joints are affected, for example, hip or knee joints. It is likely that, during severe, infection-related diarrheal diseases, the mucosal barrier of the intestine is so severely damaged that pathogens or their products enter the bloodstream. Then, antibodies can be formed against microbial components that also recognize substances of the cartilage. Such "cross-reacting" antibodies then bind to cartilage and trigger inflammations. In the case of reactive arthritis, unlike RA, the inflammation usually subsides when the pathogens are eliminated.

Very similar to reactive arthritis, components of harmless intestinal bacteria also trigger cross-reacting antibodies against similar body proteins in the joint gap in RA patients (Pianta et al. 2017). Since molecules of the microbiome often come into contact with the human immune system, it is almost banal that cross-reacting immune responses are also constantly being created. But why then do not more people get RA? Probably because, in healthy people, inflammatory responses are blocked early on by their immune tolerance. However, in people with a predisposition to RA, this brake works less well, which may have sometimes been an advantage in the past. In this context, it is interesting that, in some populations of indigenous people in North America, RA occurs in 5 to 6% of people (Peschken and Esdaile 1999). Such an accumulation—the worldwide prevalence is 0.5 to 1%—can only occur if the corresponding genes provided an advantage during evolution. Perhaps the Native Americans were protected from certain infections because their immune system responded particularly easily to microbial stimuli. However, this originally positive characteristic is reversed in today's world, where infections have become rare.

Celiac Disease

Increasing Grumbling in the Stomach

Our vacations in Sweden were often a real eye-opener for my wife and me when it came to food: Everywhere in the supermarket shelves, and even on the menus of trendy restaurants, there was an abundance of vegetarian, vegan, and gluten-free options. "Wow, no Cow," as the clever and witty advertising goes from Oatly, the brand that has made a big business out of Swedish oat milk. In restaurants, the staff proactively asks about potential allergies and has a list of the 20 most important allergens ready. Cow's milk with coffee is not a given, as soy, oat, or almond milk might also be desired. "What's gotten into the Scandinavians?" one wonders. Obviously, the sensitivity to diet-related complaints is considerably higher there than in Germany.

Returning home sensitized by the holiday experiences, one sees the same trend—with some delay. Here, too, sales of alternatives to dairy products and vegan or gluten-free foods are in high demand—especially among the younger group of buyers. In Germany, for example, the proportion of vegan products in new food introductions has risen from 1% in 2012 to 14% in 2018 (Statista 2018). Why is this? Is it a fashion phenomenon, do consumers want to save the world by abstaining from animal products, or does the increased consumption reflect the nation's stomach aches? This question is difficult to answer, as there are hardly any scientifically proven statistics. One of the examples found on the internet: The issue of the journal Ärzteblatt from June 1, 2018, quotes a study that found that, in a survey of 2000 German citizens, 25% of the participants claim to suffer from food intolerances. Women are slightly more affected than men. However, only 7% reportedly seek advice from doctors, pharmacists, or nutrition experts. So, the actual prevalence of the disease is likely to be somewhat lower than 25%, but even then, it is still surprisingly high.

Another thing that Ärzteblatt writes: Non-sufferers often have little sympathy for the stomach aches of others. They assume that a good part of the suffering is imagined. Lactose intolerance, gluten intolerance, histamine sensitivity, food allergies... The list is long, and one wonders why one "used to" hear so little about it. Did people simply ignore these ailments, brush them off with the motto "What doesn't kill me makes me stronger," or have these intolerances actually increased?

Let's take celiac disease as an example, an inflammatory disease triggered by gluten proteins from certain types of grain. A comparative Finnish study showed that the number of antibody-positive individuals in the population has doubled within two decades (Lohi et al. 2007), and another study documents a 6.4-fold increase in the incidence of celiac disease within 20 years in Scotland (White et al. 2013). So, celiac disease, like other inflammatory diseases, has increased significantly in recent decades and the "perceived increase" has a real background.

However, the multitude of different ailments, which manifest themselves in stomach rumbling and digestive problems, complicates the overview. On the one hand, there are many intolerances, in which hard-to-digest carbohydrates, such as those from vegetables, fruit, or dairy products, reach the large intestine and increase the activity of the bacteria there. Bloating, a feeling of fullness, and diarrhea are the result, but inflammation plays no role. Therefore, these intolerances are not discussed here. Also, food components that irritate the immune system, and thus enhance inflammation, are not discussed here. And food allergies, whose characteristic is the formation of IgE antibodies, have already been addressed earlier.

It becomes complicated when several components in a food simultaneously trigger different diseases, whose symptoms may even resemble each other. For example, wheat can trigger both allergies and celiac disease. In addition, the substances it contains can increase inflammatory responses, and hard-to-digest carbohydrates can cause unpleasant intestinal disorders (Schuppan and Gisbert-Schuppan 2018). However, wheat as such is not dangerous, as millions consume bread, pasta or cake with great appetite and without problems every day. Unfortunately, not everyone can tolerate gluten-containing grains, and those who are affected must avoid it. It is helpful when doctors accurately diagnose which substances in the food cause the complaints in susceptible individuals, as exact knowledge of the cause can facilitate therapy. However, due to the difficult diagnosis of digestive problems, the diagnosis of "irritable bowel syndrome" is often made, which says nothing about its causes.

Celiac Disease, the "Iceberg Disease"

Discomfort, abdominal pain, bloating and diarrhea or constipation after consuming grain products are a sign of celiac disease, or "sprue". The disease usually occurs either in childhood (first to ninth year of life) or in adulthood. The cause is gluten, the adhesive protein of various grains, which gives baked goods their elastic consistency. In some affected individuals, even small amounts of gluten trigger severe symptoms, while in others, it causes hardly any reactions, despite their illness. However, with prolonged consumption of gluten-containing foods, almost all susceptible individuals develop inflammation that causes the villi in the small intestine to recede. This causes the intestine to lose its ability to efficiently absorb nutrients, vitamins and trace elements. This leads to developmental disorders in children and causes deficiency symptoms such as anemia and osteoporosis. In women, celiac disease can lead to fertility problems, pregnancies can be complicated and the children of sick women are often underweight.

The symptoms of celiac disease can be so unspecific that even trained doctors do not think of ordering a meaningful antibody test. Thus, 80–90% of those affected have only a few symptoms that actually affect the intestine, but they experience other signs of disease (Deutsche Zöliakie-Gesellschaft 2019). Patients can live with celiac disease for years with virtually no symptoms, but, at the same time, have dangerously advanced intestinal changes. The diagnosis of such occult forms is often due to chance; therefore, the disease is sometimes referred to as the "celiac iceberg". Common symptoms include headaches, fatigue, dizziness, joint and muscle pain, and depressive moods. Skin changes can occur, manifesting as intensely itching blisters on the buttocks, knees and elbows or scalp, caused by autoimmune responses. Increasingly, however, celiac disease is also being associated with neurological disorders. The most striking of these is gluten ataxia, a movement disorder that is the result of damage to nerve cells (Caio et al. 2019). Celiac disease is therefore a disease that affects not only the intestine, but the entire body system.

The only possible treatment for celiac patients today is a lifelong, completely gluten-free diet. Even though there is now a large range of corresponding baked goods and pasta, such a diet poses a great challenge, as gluten is contained in many ready-made products. In addition, gluten-free products are significantly more expensive and not available everywhere.

Whether and how the disease develops depends on, among other things, the timing and nature of the first contact with gluten. This fact is very vividly illustrated by a Swedish study illustrating a veritable epidemic of celiac disease in toddlers. In the early 1980s, Swedish baby food manufacturers had increased the proportion of wheat, rye, and barley in children's food, but reduced the proportion of low-gluten oats. As celiac disease cases increased, the recommendation in Sweden between 1985 and 1987 was to give toddlers grain-containing food only after weaning at the age of 6 months. As a result, the number of new cases of celiac disease in children shot up fivefold. In response to the increase, the recommendations were changed in 1996: parents should now feed their children smaller amounts of grain food during breastfeeding from the fourth month. At the same time, the manufacturers of commercial children's food reduced the gluten content of their products. As a result, the number of new cases in children in Sweden returned to the initial value (Ivarsson et al. 2000).

In genetically susceptible children, the circumstances of the introduction of grain food thus influence the risk of celiac disease. Probably, feeding grain in the first months of life reduces the risk of later celiac disease, because the child's immune system can still be easily imprinted towards tolerance. This pattern is strongly reminiscent of the studies mentioned earlier on peanut allergy, which is less common in children with early allergen contact (Du Toit et al. 2015).

Just a few decades ago, celiac disease was a rare, difficult to diagnose disease that mainly occurred in children. Nowadays, there are modern antibody tests that allow for comparative studies with stored sera. Thus, in studies with sera from Air Force cadets in the USA, it was shown that the frequency of celiac disease increased fivefold between the 1950s and the 1990s (Rubio-Tapi et al. 2009). A similar increase is also observed in other industrialized countries. In Germany, such tests are now positive in about 1% of the population, but only 10–20% of these people have the full picture of the disease. In addition, however, there are 5–7% of Germans who are affected by a wheat sensitivity, whose symptoms are very similar to celiac disease. Due to the high proportion of wheat, rye, and barley in the diet, celiac disease was previously essentially limited to Western Europe and the European-descendant population of the USA (Lindfors et al. 2019). In contrast, its frequency is now increasing in the wake of the Western lifestyle, with the higher popularity of pizza and burgers in Africa and East Asia as well (Lindfors et al. 2019).

How Gluten Becomes a Problem

At the keyword "gluten", one suspects an exactly defined substance that plays a role in connection with celiac disease. Gluten, however, is a collective term for a mixture of different proteins that some types of grain store as a reserve substance in the outer layer of their seeds, the gluten layer. Wheat, rye, and barley, but also, to a lesser extent, oats, contain these proteins. Also, the precursors of wheat, such as emmer, spelt, spelled, einkorn, and kamut, contain gluten, whereas corn, rice, millet, buckwheat, and quinoa are free of it. The positive property of gluten is its rubbery, sticky consistency when it comes into contact with water. This consistency makes the gluten protein almost indispensable for bread baking, as it gives the dough its cohesion, elasticity, and juiciness. The "gluten protein" consists of a multitude of similar proteins, which are divided into different subgroups. Actually, "gluten" is a rather imprecise term.

While most proteins are broken down into individual amino acids by digestive enzymes from the stomach, pancreas, and intestinal cells, gluten, due to its complex structure, is difficult to digest and is often only broken down into fragments. Such fragments can enter the body's interior when the intestinal barrier is damaged and encounter phagocytes there. These garbage collectors take up the fragments and break them down into even smaller pieces. An important change occurs in the process: The enzyme transglutaminase of the phagocytes alters individual amino acids of the fragments, creating new structures that the immune system recognizes well. In some people, such altered gluten fragments are now very efficiently presented by phagocytes to the T cells of the immune system (Reif and Lerner 2004).

T cells that recognize the altered gluten fragments well are activated, divide, and their offspring release inflammation-promoting cytokines, with which they attract and activate other immune cells. These newcomers release aggressive molecules, damaging the surrounding tissue and attracting more cells. The resulting inflammation stresses the intestinal epithelial cells, which then begin to produce cytokines themselves. Among other things, they release IL-15, a cytokine that inhibits regulatory T cells, and thus blocks an important immune brake. Often, these processes also lead to an increased permeability of the intestinal barrier, so that more gluten fragments encounter phagocytes, escalating the reaction. Without a supply of gluten, the inflammation usually subsides and fully regresses. Only in a small fraction of patients with "recurrent celiac disease" do the inflammation and associated intestinal changes persist even after discontinuing gluten-containing food (Lindfors et al. 2019).

Antibodies directed against the body's own enzyme transglutaminase are also involved in the development of the disease. Thus, celiac disease also has an autoimmune component. These antibodies in particular accumulate in the endomysium, a sheath that surrounds individual muscle bundles of the smooth muscle. These antibodies can damage the muscle. However, recent publications also report effects of the antibodies on the brain. There, according to these studies, damage occurred in the cerebellum in a few patients, leading to movement, speech, and coordination disorders ("gluten ataxia"). Other neurological diseases are also associated with celiac disease (Pennisi et al. 2017).

Celiac disease affects individuals whose immune system recognizes the enzymatically altered gluten peptides well. In this recognition, the proteins of the HLA system, which present protein fragments to T cells on the surface of phagocytes, play a crucial role. Over 90% of celiac patients have HLA genes of type DQ2, which are thus the most important risk genes for celiac disease. However, the disease must have additional causes, as about 40% of the European-descendant population carries these genes and the majority of these people are healthy. In addition to the HLA genes, more than 40 other risk genes are found in celiac disease. Many of these gene variants influence the immune response and also occur in other inflammatory diseases, showing the common roots of these ailments. In addition, triggering factors are suspected that are not yet precisely known. And this is where the microbiome comes into play again.

The Role of the Microbiome in Celiac Disease

Epidemiological studies, some of which were supported by laboratory experiments and animal model studies, attribute a role as a trigger of celiac disease to intestinal infections with certain viruses, which were previously considered relatively harmless. For example, the reovirus, once known as essentially innocuous, is now suspected of reprogramming the immune system towards inflammatory responses and loss of tolerance (Bouziat et al. 2017), and infections with rotaviruses could also trigger celiac disease (Meijer et al. 2018). Apparently, pathogens can also reduce the risk of disease. So, for example, it has been observed that celiac disease occurs less frequently in people infected with the stomach bacterium Helicobacter pylori than would be expected based on genetic risk (Lerner 2017). This effect could be due to the potentially dangerous pathogen—according to the hygiene hypothesis—bringing a positive side effect in the form of an inflammation brake.

In celiac disease, similar to other inflammatory diseases, an imbalanced gut flora with reduced species diversity is observed. Studies with children also show a reduced number of anti-inflammatory bacteria, for example, of bifidobacteria (Meijer et al. 2018). There is also speculation that celiac disease could be partly caused by the loss of bacterial species that break down the difficult-to-digest gluten protein in the intestine. Such bacteria are apparently not uncommon. Spanish scientists isolated almost 100 bacterial strains from stool samples that could break down gluten. Some of these strains also broke down a specific gluten fragment that causes problems for most celiac patients and triggers autoimmune responses (Caminero et al. 2014). An enzyme that digests gluten has now even been isolated from a commensal bacterium in the oral cavity (Wei et al. 2020). Therefore, a suitable gut flora could possibly reduce the gluten load, and thus the likelihood of disease. In the future, targeted colonization with probiotic bacteria that break down gluten could even prevent the development of celiac disease (Fig. 5.8).

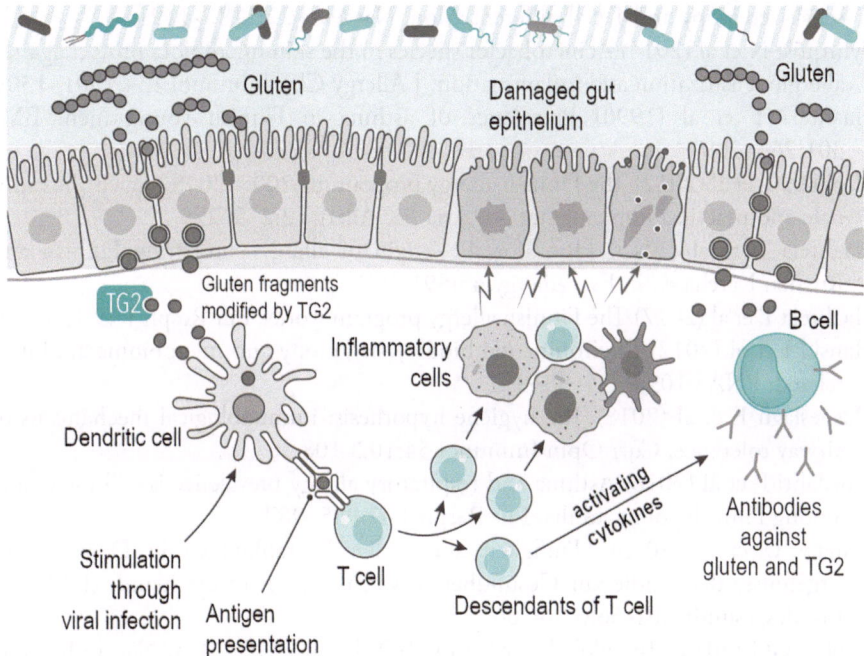

Fig. 5.8 Development of celiac disease. Fragments of gluten pass through the intestinal epithelium and are altered by transglutaminase (TG2). Presentation by phagocytes induces T cells, whose offspring attract inflammatory cells with their cytokines. The inflammation damages the intestinal epithelium. At the same time, antibodies against gluten and TG2 are also formed, which contribute to the disease. (© Scorpio Verlag in Europa Verlage GmbH, München. Reproduced with permission)

References

Allergic Diseases

Ansaldo E (2021) Control of immunity by the microbiota. Ann Rev Immunol 39:449–479

Bergmann KC et al (2016) Aktueller Stand zur Verbreitung von Allergien in Deutschland. Allergo J Int 25:6–10

DGAKI/DGKJ (2014) S3-Leitlinien https://www.awmf.org/guidelines/detail/ll/061-016.html. Accessed 1 Mar 2022

Du Toit G et al (2008) Early consumption of peanuts in infancy is associated with a low prevalence of peanut allergy. J Allergy Clin Immunol 122:984–991

Du Toit G et al (2015) Randomized trial of peanut consumption in infants at risk for peanut allergy. N Engl J Med 372:803–813

EEACI (2018) Advocacy manifesto. Tackling the allergy crisis in Europe–concerted policy action needed. https://www.eaaci.org/outreach.html. Accessed 1 Mar 2022

Fujimori KE et al (2016) Neonatal gut microbiota associates with childhood multi-sensitized atopy and T cell differentiation. Nat Med 22:1187–1191

Fyhrquist N et al (2014) Acinetobacter species in the skin microbiota protect against allergic sensitization and inflammation. J Allergy Clin Immunol 134:1301–1309

Haahtela T et al (1990) Prevalence of asthma in Finnish young men. BMJ 301:266–268

Haahtela T et al (2012) The Finnish allergy programme 2008–2018 – scientific rationale and practical implementation. Asia Pac Allergy 2:275–279

Haahtela T et al (2015) Hunt for the origin of allergy–comparing Finnish and Russian Karelia. Clin Exp Allergy 45:891–901

Haahtela T et al (2017) The Finnish allergy program works. Eur Respir J 49:1700470

Hanski I et al (2012) Environmental biodiversity, atopy and microbiome are inter-related. PNAS 109:8334–8339

Haspeslagh E et al (2018) The hygiene hypothesis: immunological mechanisms of airway tolerance. Curr Opin Immunol 54:102–108

Jousilahti P et al (2016) Asthma and respiratory allergy prevalence is still increasing among Finnish young adults. Eur Respir J 47:985–987

Langen U et al (2013) Häufigkeit allergischer Erkrankungen in Deutschland. Ergebnisse der Studie zur Gesundheit Erwachsener in Deutschland. (DEGS1). Bundesgesundheitsb 56:698–706

Kaplan GG (2015) The global burden of IBD: From 2015–2025. Nature Reviews Gastroenterol. Hepatol 12:720–727

Machiels K et al (2014) A decrease of the butyrate-producing species Roseburia hominis and Faecalibacterium prausnitzii defines dysbiosis in patients with ulcerative colitis. Gut 63:1275–1283

Platts-Mills TAE (2015) The allergy epidemics: 1870–2010. J Allergy Clin Immunol 136:3–13

Roduit C et al (2018) High levels of butyrate and propionate in early life are associated with protection against allergy. Allergy 74:799–809

Roslund MI et al (2020) Biodiversity intervention enhances immune regulation and health-associated commensal microbiota among day-care children. Sci Adv 6:eaba2578

Ruokolainen L et al (2015) Green areas around homes reduce atopic sensitization in children. Eur J Allergy Clin Immunol 70:195–202

To T et al (2012) Global asthma prevalence in adults: findings from the cross sectional world health survey. BMC Public Health 12:204

Tyagi N et al (2015) Comparison of allergenic and metazoan parasite proteins: allergy the price of immunity. PLoS Comp Biol 11:e1004546

Weidiger S, Novak N (2016) Atopic dermatitis. Lancet 387:1109–1122

Williams H et al (2016) Is eczema really on the increase worldwide? J Allergy Clin Immunol 121:947–954

Chronic Inflammatory Bowel Diseases (IBD)

Burisch J, Munkholm P (2015) The epidemiology of inflammatory bowel disease. Scand J Gastroenterol 50:942–951

Burisch J et al (2014) West-east gradient of IBD in Europe: the ECCO-EpiCom inception cohort. Gut 63:588–597

Degenhardt F, Franke A (2017) Genetics of Crohn's disease and ulcerative colitis. Gastroenterologe 1:38–48

Fukui H (2016) Increased intestinal permeability and decreased barrier function: does it really influence the risk of inflammation? Inflamm Intest Dis 1:135–145

Halfvarson J et al (2017) Dynamics of the human microbiome in inflammatory bowel disease. Nat Microbiol 2:17004

Hammer T et al (2016) The Faroese IBD study. Incidence of inflammatory bowel diseases across 54 years of population-based data. J Crohns Colitis 10:934–942

Hammer T et al (2017) Inflammatory bowel diseases in Faroese-born Danish residents and their offspring: further evidence of the dominant role of environmental factors in IBD development. Aliment Pharmacol Ther 45:1107–1114

Hammer T et al (2019) Dietary risk factors for inflammatory bowel diseases in a high-risk population: results from the Faroese IBD study. United Eur Gastroenterol J 7:924–932

Kedia S, Ahuja V (2017) Epidemiology of IBD in India: the great shift east. Inflamm Dis 2:102–115

Loftus EV (2004) Clinical epidemiology of inflammatory bowel disease: incidence, prevalence, and environmental influences. Gastroenterol 126:1504–1517

Mulder DJ et al (2014) A tale of two diseases: the history of inflammatory bowel diseases. J Crohns Colitis 8:341–348

Ng SC et al (2017) Worldwide incidence and prevalence of inflammatory bowel disease in the 21st century: a systematic review of population-based studies. Lancet 390:2769–2778

Rizzello F et al (2019) Implications of the westernized diet in the onset and progression of IBD. Nutrients 11:1033

Sellon RK et al (1998) Resident enteric bacteria are necessary for development of spontaneous colitis and immune system activation in interleukin-10-deficient mice. Infect Immun 66:5224–5231

Vavricka SR et al (2015) Extraintestinal manifestations of inflammatory bowel disease. Am J Gastroenterol 106:110–119

Virta LJ et al (2017) IBD on the rise in Finland, except for the very young. J Crohns Colitis 11:150–156

Type 1 Diabetes (T1D)

Bason C et al (2013) In type 1 diabetes a subset of anti-Coxsackie-virus B4 antibodies recognize autoantigens and induce apoptosis of pancreatic beta cells. PLoS One 8:e57729

Harjutsalo V et al (2008) Time trends in the incidence of type1 diabetes in Finnish children: a cohort study. Lancet 71:1777–1782

Kent SC (2017) Deciphering the pathogenesis of human type 1 diabetes (T1D) by interrogating T cells from the "scene of the crime". Curr Diab Rep 17:95

Marfil-Garza BA et al (2020) Progress in translational regulatory T cell therapies for type 1 diabetes and islet transplantation. Endocr Rev 15:198–218

Miettinen ME et al (2020) Serum 25-hydroxyvitamin D concentration in childhood and risk of islet autoimmunity and type 1 diabetes: the TRIGR nested case–control ancillary study. Diabetologia 63:780–787

Niinistö S et al (2017) Fatty acid status in infancy is associated with the risk of type 1 diabetes-associated autoimmunity. Diabetologia 60:1223–1233

Patterson CC et al (2019) Trends and cyclical variation in the incidence of childhood type 1 diabetes in 26 European centres in the 25 year period 1989–2013: a multicentre prospective registration study. Diabetologia 62:408–417

Pociot A, Lermark A (2016) Type 1 diabetes series: genetic risk factors for type 1 diabetes. Lancet 387:2331–2339

Siljander H et al (2019) Microbiome and type 1 diabetes. EBio Med 46:512–521

Thomaidou S et al (2018) Islet stress, degradation and autoimmunity. Diabetes Obes Metab 20:88–94

Vatanen T et al (2016) Variation in microbiome LPS immunogenicity contributes to autoimmunity in humans. Cell 165:842–853

Multiple Sclerosis (MS)

Berer K et al (2017) Gut microbiota from MS patients enables spontaneous encepha-lomyelitis in mice. PNAS 114:10729–10724

Cekanaviciute E et al (2017) Gut bacteria from MS patients modulate human T cells and exacerbate symptoms in mouse models. PNAS 114:10713–10718

Chen J et al (2016a) MS patients have a distinct gut microbiota compared to healthy controls. Sci Rep 6:28484

Dobson R, Giovannoni G (2019) Multiple sclerosis – a review. Eur J Neurol 26:27–40

Filippi M et al (2018) Multiple sclerosis. Nat Rev Dis Primers 4:43

Hollenbach JA, Oksenberg JR (2015) The immunogenetics of MS. J Autoimmun 64:13–25

Jangi S et al (2016) Alterations of the human gut microbiome in MS. Nat Commun 7:12015

Kingwell E et al (2013) Incidence and prevalence of MS in Europe: a systematic review. BMC Neurol 13:128

Koch-Henriksen N, Soerensen PS (2010) The changing demographic pattern in MS epidemiology. Lancet Neurol 9:520–532

MS International Federation (2020). https://www.msif.org. Accessed 4 Mar 2021

Planas R et al (2018) GDP-L-fucose synthase is a CD4+ specific auto-antigen in DRB3*02:02 patients with MS. Sci Trans Med 10:eaat4301

Wendel-Haga M, Celius EG (2017) Is the hygiene hypothesis relevant for the risk of multiple sclerosis? Acta Neurol Scand 136(Suppl 201):36–30

Psoriasis

Benhadou F et al (2019) Psoriasis: keratinocytes or immune cells – which is the trig-ger? Dermatology 235:91–100

Gibbs S (1996) Skin disease and socioeconomic conditions in rural Africa: Tanzania. Int J Dermatol 35(9):633–639

Greb JE et al (2016) Psoriasis. Nat Rev Dis Primers 2:16082

Kunz M et al (2019) Psoriasis: obesity and fatty acids. Trends Immunol 10:1807

Yunusbaeva M et al (2018) Psoriasis patients demonstrate HLA-Cw*06:02 allele dos-age dependent T cell proliferation when treated with hair follicle-derived keratin 17 protein. Sci Rep 8:6098

Rheumatoid Arthritis (RA)

Chen J et al (2016b) An expansion of rare lineage intestinal microbes characterizes rheumatoid arthritis. Genome Med 8:43

Dixon WG (2019) How the weather affects the pain of citizen scientists using a smartphone app. Digit Med 2:105

Kallberg H et al (2011) Smoking is a major preventable risk factor for rheumatoid arthritis: estimations of risks after various exposures to cigarette smoke. Ann Rheum Dis 70:508–511

Lefèvre S et al (2009) Synovial fibroblasts spread rheumatoid arthritis to unaffected joints. Nat Med 15:1414–1420

Peschken CA, Esdaile JM (1999) Rheumatic diseases in North America's indigenous peoples. Sem Arthr Rheum 28:368–369

Pianta A et al (2017) Two rheumatoid arthritis–specific autoantigens correlate microbial immunity with autoimmune responses in joints. J Clin Invest 127:2946–2956

Smolen JS et al (2018) Rheumatoid arthritis. Nat Rev Dis Primers 4:18001

Celiac Disease

Bouziat R et al (2017) Reovirus infection triggers inflammatory responses to dietary antigens and development of celiac disease. Science 356:44–50

Caio G et al (2019) Celiac disease: a comprehensive current review. BMC Med 17:142–162

Caminero A et al (2014) Diversity of the cultivable human gut microbiome involved in gluten metabolism: isolation of microorganisms with potential interest for celiac disease. FEMS Microbiol Ecol 88:309–319

Deutsche Zöliakie-Gesellschaft (2019). https://www.dzg-online.de/homepage.1.0.html. Accessed 27 Jan 2019

Du Toit G (2015) Randomized trial of peanut consumption in infants at risk for peanut allergy. N Engl J Med 372:803–813

Ivarsson A et al (2000) Epidemic of celiac disease in Swedish children. Acta Paediatr 89(165):71

Lerner A (2017) Microbes and viruses are bugging the gut in celiac disease. Front Microbiol 8:1392

Lindfors K et al (2019) Celiac disease. Nat Rev Dis Primers 5:3

Lohi S et al (2007) Increasing prevalence of celiac disease over time. Aliment Pharmacol Ther 26:1217–1225

Meijer C et al (2018) Celiac disease prevention. Front Pediatr 6:368

Pennisi M et al (2017) Neurophysiology of the "celiac brain": disentangling gut-brain connections. Front Neurosci 11:498

Reif S, Lerner A (2004) Tissue transglutaminase – the key player in celiac disease: a review. Autoimmun Rev 3:40–45

Rubio-Tapi A et al (2009) Increased prevalence and mortality in undiagnosed celiac disease. Gastroenterology 137:373–374

Schuppan D, Gisbert-Schuppan K (2018) Tägliches Brot: Krank durch Weizen, Gluten und ATI. Springer, Heidelberg

Statista   (2018).   https://de.statista.com/statistik/daten/studie/692158/umfrage/
  Anteil-veganer-Lebensmittel-bei-Produktionsneueinführung-in-Deutschland.
  Accessed 2 Mar 2022
Wei G et al (2020) Commensal bacterium Rothia aeria degrades and detoxifies glu-
  ten via a highly effective subtilisin enzyme. Nutrients 12:3724
White LE et al (2013) The rising incidence of celiac disease in Scotland. Pediatrics
  132:e924–e931

6

Food for the Superorganism

Contents

Grandma's Kitchen

On our kitchen shelf, in a prominent place, sits the "Great Illustrated Edition for the Civil and Fine Cuisine" of the Kiehnle Cookbook. First published in 1912 by Hermine Kiehnle, the head of a Swabian cooking school, it has now been published over a million times in various revisions, and is still sold today. Our 1927 edition conveys the collected kitchen wisdom of the time through "2085 tested recipes". In addition to recipes for every conceivable dish, it suggests weekly menus and festive meals and gives advice for meatless cooking and sick meals. It even explains in detail how to keep the kitchen clean.

The special thing: Whether it was pasta, dumplings, mayonnaise, jam or goose liver pate, everything was made from fresh, basic ingredients. Grandma's kitchen knew no ready-made pizza and there were no Asian noodle dishes to boil. There was no frozen food or microwave, and canned goods were a rarity. Even today, there are cooking fans who have the same ambition, and everything they produce is "homemade". But the vast majority either starts with pre-made products or buys ready-made meals that require little work. With this modern way of eating, there is a risk of stressing your microbiome and promoting the development of inflammatory diseases.

Through evolution, humans, including the modern city dweller, are actually optimized for a life as hunters and gatherers. The length of our intestines, which lies between that of carnivores and herbivores, indicates a mixed diet. Nutritional physiology says that we have an enormously flexible digestive system that can adapt to the most diverse diets. From the Inuit in Greenland, who originally lived almost exclusively on meat and bacon, to Indian vegetarians: We can adapt, and this is certainly to a large part due to our microbiome. It is probably correct to assume that our early ancestors' diet was similar to that of today's hunters and gatherers. Their diet is largely plant-based and consists mostly of tubers, fruits, leaves, seeds, and nuts. Meat is available when the season and hunting luck provide game.

About 10,000 years ago, a climate change altered living conditions so that agriculture became possible, with most human societies switching to farming and livestock breeding. This "Neolithic Revolution" could be called the first dietary revolution, because, from then on, grain products dominated the diet. The new, grain-based food was not necessarily better, but it fed more people, and therefore became a successful model. This change seems to have been relatively well tolerated by humans, because, in traditional societies that still mainly live on grain, inflammatory diseases are virtually unknown. These ailments, such as allergies, asthma, and chronic intestinal inflammation, became more widespread in industrialized countries after the Second World War. Their increase went hand in hand with a change in the food systems, which was so drastic that one could speak of a second dietary revolution.

An important feature of this second dietary revolution is the abandonment of self-sufficiency with food from one's own garden or field and the departure from self-made food. A food industry emerged that largely relieved people of the need to produce their own food. With its products, it made everyday life easier, but, at the same time, also created new trends and developed modern foods with innovative techniques, which are often far away from natural food. Some of the products that emerged would probably be rejected with horror by Hermine Kiehnle. Made from a narrow range of the cheapest pre-made products and spiced up with sugar, salt, and flavorings; preserved and shaped with preservatives and emulsifiers. The essential point, however, is that, in this artificial diet, the nutrients are present in a different way than they are in natural products, and they are digested differently. Those who want to delve deeper into this can find information on the structure and properties of carbohydrates, fats, proteins, and micronutrients (vitamins, minerals, secondary plant substances) in the "Macro and Micronutrients" section in Chap. 8.

This artificial diet is a strain on our inner ecosystem for many reasons. Why? Like an over-fertilized lawn, it promotes the growth of fewer species at the expense of species diversity, supports harmful bacteria, and thus contributes to the development of inflammatory diseases. A return to home-cooked food could help to bring our bacterial inner life back into balance. Hermine Kiehnle's cookbook would be a good companion on this journey.

Modern Foods

Were we to seek out the exact opposite of Hermine Kiehnle's home-cooked Swabian specialties from 1912, we would find the creations of modern food technology that fill supermarket shelves today. Fast food, soft drinks, and prepackaged foods, like instant soups, chicken nuggets, or pudding, industrially produced from mostly cheap basic ingredients, enriched with additives and spruced up with artificial flavors, are on the rise worldwide. Many of the foods that are commonplace today were virtually unknown about 50 years ago, before the onset of the allergy epidemic. Frozen pizza, ready-made pasta from the refrigerated section, or microwave meals did not exist! These foods are now industrial products like cars or furniture. They must, above all, be easy to produce, inexpensive, and have a good shelf life. To sell well, they must, of course, also appeal to the consumer in taste and appearance. In addition to shape and color, properties such as spreadability or the ability to melt in the mouth are optimized. This can be achieved through various additives. These artificial products certainly meet the legal requirements, but are they also healthy?

A prime example of these modern foods are chips: Once found mainly in the form of potato chips, a rather boring accompaniment to evenings in front of the television, they are now available in so many flavors, textures, colors and aromas that there is always something new to discover. Even the eating experience is taken into account, for example, the stability of potato or corn chips is calculated exactly so that they break with a certain pressure from the tongue, the sound of which gives us pleasure. No wonder that about 40% of Germans over 14 years old reach for chips several times a month. The same is true for other industrial products that are full of sugar or fat, such as Peanut flips, chocolate, nut nougat cream, cookies and cream cakes. But ready-made pizza, fatty burgers, frozen meals, ice cream and desserts are also similarly tempting. The more you consume, the more dangerous belly fat grows and the risk of heart attack, stroke and type 2 diabetes, but also of inflammatory diseases, increases.

The secret of the popularity of highly processed foods is once again revealed through the lens of evolution, which always calculates for times of need. The body prepares as if the next famine winter were at the door. Fat and sugar can be easily converted into belly fat, so our reward centers respond to these substances and we develop a preference for them that borders on addiction. Never in the history of humankind has so much sugar been consumed as is today! A particularly strong kick is triggered by a combination of fat and sugar in a mixing ratio of about 35:50. Foods that are knitted according to this "eating formula" are irresistible to us (Hoch et al. 2015). This mix puts the brain in such a high mood that satiety signals are overrun, and you continue to eat. Rats eat 30% more calories with this superfood than they would normally consume (Hoch et al. 2013).

Humans work in a very similar way: Whoops, the whole bar of chocolate is gone, even though you had planned to nibble only a single piece. "Hedonic hyperphagia" (lat.: about lustful overeating) is the scientific name of this state. Many modern foods have such an effect, being quasi-addictive and promoting obesity, especially in children (Santos-Costa et al. 2017). We also have an unhealthy preference for salt, because it was scarce in ancient times. The body does not pay attention to the fact that too much salt is unhealthy and, besides high blood pressure, also fuels inflammatory processes in the intestine, so that dormant chronic intestinal inflammations can flare up again (Marion-Letellier et al. 2019). Anyone who wants to sell their products does well to rely on the incentives of evolution. The food industry has understood this lesson.

A characteristic of modern artificial food is the high degree of processing. It is usually not made from grains, fruits or vegetables, but from basic materials such as starch, sugar, proteins or vegetable oils. In addition, there are preservatives, emulsifiers, defoamers, thickeners, flavors and other additives. The production often involves high temperatures and pressures, which is why they are referred to in English technical language as "processed food" or, even more memorably, "ultra processed food". The German term "highly processed foods" is still somewhat unfamiliar; "junk food" trips more easily off the tongue. In many of these modern products, the nutrients such as sugar, starch or fat are densely packed and lack fiber. The nutrients from these calorie-dense foods are mainly absorbed in the small intestine, but make the bacteria in the large intestine unemployed. They then necessarily attack the intestinal mucosa.

But it's not just the components like fat, sugar, or salt that make up modern food. A significant difference in artificial food: The nutrients are very easily accessible to the digestive system. They are not—as with many plant foods—enclosed in plant cells, whose walls must first be cracked by bacteria. From cooked and finely ground plant pulp, which was pressed through tiny nozzles at high pressure, the body can extract nutrients much more easily than from original plant tissue. Therefore, there is often a difference in terms of accessible calories between highly processed and natural foods. A whole grain roll does not provide nearly as much energy as a white flour roll of the same weight, explains nutrition specialist Michael Blaut, professor at the German Institute for Nutritional Research in Potsdam. With whole grain flour, some of the nutrients are still enclosed in plant cells and are only released in the large intestine, where the cells are dissolved by bacteria. However, hardly any nutrients are absorbed into the body there, but they do benefit bacteria that would starve with white flour.

This easy accessibility of nutrients in highly processed foods also has other consequences that are hardly known to the layman. Andreas Pfeiffer, Professor of Endocrinology and Metabolic Medicine at the Berlin Charité, explained to me: With easily available calories, as they are present in typical highly processed food, the majority of nutrients are quickly absorbed in the upper part of the small intestine. In particular, sugars, which either come directly from the food or are produced by splitting starch, enter the blood there and stimulate the production of the hormone GIP (glucose dependent insulinotropic polypeptide). This messenger substance causes a redirection of calories into fat storage, and thus leads to obesity, which, in turn, promotes inflammation. However, these calories do not cause a pronounced feeling of satiety. This mainly occurs when nutrients from complex food are absorbed in the lower part of the small intestine. This stimulates the production of the hormone GLP1 (glucagon-like peptide 1), which conveys a feeling of satiety and ensures that the food is retained in the stomach for longer. So, the greater the proportion of highly processed food with easily accessible nutrients, the more calories are immediately shifted into fat storage, without satiety and a feeling of fullness setting in. Therefore, easily digestible fast food does not leave as lasting a feeling of satiety as natural food, but is more noticeable on the scales. Similarly, calorie-rich sugar sodas hardly satiate, although they flood the body with calories.

Modern artificial food can therefore leave a feeling of hunger despite a sufficient amount of calories, which encourages further eating. However, we are not adjusted to this abundance, and so the small intestine, when too much easily digestible replenishment comes, passes the surplus on to the large intestine. There, the nutrients then lead to the growth of bacterial species that otherwise lead a shadowy existence.

As with an algal bloom in waters, certain populations then explode, while the normal large intestine bacteria, which break down plant fibers and cells and produce short-chain fatty acids from them fall behind (Zinöcker and Lindseth 2018). But these short-chain fatty acids are important for calming the immune system and slowing down the tendency to inflammatory responses. Also, the addition of emulsifiers, artificial sweeteners, flavors, salt, and other components that are supposed to make snacks, ready-to-eat meals, and cheap pastries attractive can have a strong impact on the balance among the gut bacteria.

The consumption of these highly processed foods is constantly increasing. As a concrete example, let's take Sweden: The market share of highly processed foods increased by 142% between 1960 and 2010. The largest increase was in sugary drinks, by 315%, which corresponds to an increase from 22 to 92 liters per person per year, only surpassed by snacks and sweets, whose consumption increased by 367%, or from 7 to 34 kg per person per year (Juul et al. 2015). A particular problem with these much-loved sweets and soft drinks: they contain many calories, but few micronutrients, such as vitamins, minerals, trace elements, and secondary plant substances. These "empty calories" can lead to a deficiency of micronutrients, and thus to increased susceptibility to disease. But nobody seems to care so long as junk food continues to bring in fantastic profit margins!

Many studies show the correlation between the consumption of highly processed foods and an increased risk of obesity and other dietary diseases (Zinöcker and Lindseth 2018; Beslay et al. 2020). What science painstakingly captures in exact numbers is also clear to the average person: how quickly one can increase their weight and drive up their poor blood values with a burger and cola-based "modern" diet is very impressively demonstrated by documentaries such as the American film "Supersize Me", which can be found on YouTube. Even though the action in this case takes place in the USA, the reality has long since arrived in Europe: In a French study of 44,000 people, conducted at the Sorbonne in Paris, the proportion of highly processed foods in the participants' calorie needs was 29% (Schnabel et al. 2019), while in Germany, this value is about 45%. We are not far away from the USA, where, on average, almost 60% of the calorie requirement is covered by highly processed foods (Baraldi et al. 2018).

This change in dietary behavior is also reflected in the statistics: In Germany, two-thirds of men and half of women are overweight; and about a quarter of adults is one step further, namely, obese (RKI 2014). Worldwide, in 2017, almost one in three, namely, 2.4 billion people, was overweight, with greatly increased risks for cardiovascular diseases, type 2 diabetes and inflammatory diseases (GBD 2017, Diet Collaborators 2019). Especially among children, the number of obese individuals has massively increased in the last four decades, by tenfold! (WHO 2017).

At the same time, these over-nourished individuals often suffer from a lack of micronutrients, so that we speak of "hidden hunger". This malnutrition is also one of the reasons why, in some developed countries, the average life expectancy of people has recently stopped rising and begun falling (Ho and Hendi 2018). Therefore, one cannot say that the artificial diet is toxic, but it is life-shortening. A labeling requirement, accompanied by increased taxes for these products, would be desirable. The proceeds could be used to correspondingly reduce the price of healthy foods.

Of course, the unhealthy diet particularly affects low-income individuals, as the mass-produced, highly processed foods are much cheaper than corresponding fresh products. They are sufficient to eliminate the calorie deficiency, but are bad for one's health. The aforementioned French study shows that highly processed foods are consumed in poorer strata particularly by young people with low education. This cements the inequalities in society: those who are poorer and less educated than the average population eat more fast food, are more likely to get sick, and die earlier (Schnabel et al. 2019). This unequal distribution is certainly not limited to France, but can be found in any place where discount stores and organic supermarkets coexist.

Bread as an Example

Often, the differences between an industrially and a traditionally produced food are so fluid that it is difficult to pin them down. Of course, the ingredients play a big role, but the processing can also make a significant difference. These nuances can be very well illustrated with bread. What is a healthily produced bread, and what is a turbo-produced bread—a source of bloating and stomach pain, brought up to speed with chemical tricks in no time at all? Is it the crust, the color, the scent or the taste that make the difference? Thanks to food technology, all these properties can be influenced, but what constitutes real quality?

Germany is rightly proud of its traditional baking culture, which, according to the German Bread Institute, has produced almost 3200 different types of bread and is even registered as an immaterial UNESCO World Heritage. The list ranges from A to Z, namely, from "Abendbrot" (evening bread) to "Zypernbrot" (Cyprus bread) (see www.brotexperte.de). What a wealth of variations of crust and crumb! Strict legal regulations ensure that everything is in order. Bread consists essentially of four ingredients, namely, flour, water, salt and leavening agents. In addition, loaves of bread may contain various additives: Emulsifiers to improve the gas retention, the volume development and the softness of the bread. Guar gum and locust bean gum to increase the water holding capacity, and ascorbic acid to acidify the dough. Enzymes accelerate the maturation of the dough, but are then destroyed by the heating of the bread during baking, so they do not reach the consumer.

These possible ingredients, which a traditional baker will not necessarily use because of their costs, are not necessarily questionable. For example, the term ascorbic acid hides the fact that it is vitamin C, and lecithin, used as an emulsifier, is a component that is found in egg yolk and in plant seeds in larger quantities (although there are also unpleasant alternatives). Colorants and preservatives are prohibited in loaves of bread. Bread and rolls therefore do not contain the entire list of about 320 food additives allowed in the EU, even if relevant websites warn against them. But do we need additives for baking bread at all? Apparently not, because the Federal Center for Nutrition, an institution of the Federal Ministry for Nutrition and Agriculture, dryly states: "However, it is also possible to produce bread without additives." With loaves of bread, the regulations are relatively restrictive. The rules for packaged sliced bread, which may contain preservatives and anti-mold agents, are somewhat looser.

If you follow press reports, however, you will find that, apparently, more and more people are having trouble digesting baked goods. The reputation of our most important food has suffered greatly in recent years. According to recent narratives, bread doesn't only cause digestive problems, but also makes you fat, tired and sluggish. Wheat in particular is singled out as the culprit. Books like "Wheat Belly" or "Grain Brain" have stirred up the topic, and now, between 10% and 15% of the population claim to have problems digesting bread. Gluten is often blamed for this, the adhesive protein that gives bread its structure and is particularly important for the ability to bake wheat. Since media stars like actress Gwyneth Paltrow have been promoting gluten-free diets, the consumption of such foods has multiplied. However, only about 1% of Germans suffer from celiac disease, a hereditary intolerance to gluten. For most people who have to avoid bread, therefore, other causes play a role. In the past, they were often considered oversensitive, but in the last decade, thanks to intensive research, it has been found that, in addition to gluten, there are a number of other grain ingredients that can cause digestive problems and lead to inflammation.

In addition to wheat allergy, there is wheat sensitivity (or "non-celiac gluten sensitivity", NCGS), which is partly caused by natural components of the grain that protect it from insect damage. These substances block certain enzymes, but can also activate the innate immune response of humans. Some dietary fibers, the FODMAPS (fermentable oligo, di, monosaccharides and polyols), can cause abdominal pain, constipation, diarrhea, bloating or systemic complaints such as headaches or fatigue in sensitive individuals. FODMAPS have received a lot of attention in recent years, especially in connection with irritable bowel syndrome. Although dietary fibers have a positive effect as food for the bacteria of the large intestine, certain substances can activate the intestinal flora too strongly, and therefore cause problems in sensitive individuals.

This applies to whole grain bread as well as to bread made from white flour. Both flours consist mostly of starch, but also contain a proportion of positively acting dietary fibers, the ß-glucans. The difference is that, in white flour, the oil and protein-containing parts of the plant embryo, which is ready to start in the grain, and some of the dietary fibers from the outer layer of the grain are removed by repeated grinding processes. This makes white flour more durable, but it also causes it to be digested faster. During the digestion of whole grain products, the ingredients are released more slowly due to the higher proportion of dietary fibers, and they satisfy better. In addition, the dietary fibers promote the growth of intestinal bacteria, which calm the immune system with short-chain fatty acids and other metabolic products.

In view of the great interest in grain intolerance, it is being scientifically examined how the ingredients and the manufacturing processes affect the final product. The mere fact that the dough must be "machine-suitable" for industrial production requires certain additives. However, studies show that the tolerance of bread often depends less on such substances than on the manufacturing process. Especially with industrially produced bread, the aim is to shorten the production process. A lot of time can be saved during the "dough rest". All dough must "rise", meaning the contained bacteria and yeasts ferment carbohydrates and produce gases that increase the volume. This makes the bread nice and fluffy. At the same time, the microorganisms and natural active ingredients contained in the dough break down proteins (for example, enzyme inhibitors) and dietary fibers (such as the notorious FODMAPS) during the dough rest, produce digestible substances from them and also release flavorings. The dough rest is therefore a very active time, and the microorganisms in the sourdough are very efficient in breaking down complex carbohydrates.

An extended dough rest with sourdough makes the bread more digestible, but, compared to the quick baking process, it requires more time, and thus space to store the dough. For example, the production of a three-stage sourdough, which is the basis for a delicious rye mixed bread, takes 3 days. During this time, the microbes transform the flour into a nutritious food. The fifth ingredient for bread is therefore "time"! It's no wonder that bakers say "time brings flavor".

However, with permitted additives, bread can also be produced in a few hours. In many cases, pre-made baking mixes are prepared, rest for a short time and are then processed into dough pieces, which are stored frozen and baked by supermarket staff. In the short time, certain proteins and dietary fibers are not completely broken down and can cause allergic reactions, activate the innate immune system or cause bloating. These properties of conveyor belt bread are not visible, but can be felt. According to experts, the digestibility of bread could be improved solely by extending the dough resting time. The biochemist and physician Detlev Schuppan, head of the Institute for Translational Immunology at the University of Mainz, presents these correlations very convincingly in a book (Schuppan and Gisbert-Schuppan 2018).

An often-suspected cause for the poorer tolerance of modern grain products, in addition to the rapid baking processes, is the use of newly bred or possibly genetically modified grain varieties, which would have a higher content of gluten and other proteins. Especially if these components were not broken down due to shortened dough resting time and faster baking process, such produced bread could lead to discomfort. However, these rumors are not true. Apart from the fact that genetically modified grain varieties are not permitted in the EU, extensive investigations have shown that modern wheat varieties do not have a higher protein content than old varieties. On the contrary, modern wheat has a lower protein content than its ancestors Emmer, Spelt and Einkorn. The content of FODMAPS in modern wheat varieties is also no higher than in traditional ones (Longin et al. 2020; Ziegler et al. 2016; Geisslitz et al. 2019), as Prof. Friedrich Longin, a grain breeding expert from the University of Hohenheim, explained to me in an interview. The stomach pains after enjoying rolls are therefore not due to the wheat breeders, but have other causes.

Anyone who buys packaged toast from the supermarket with a minimum shelf life of 6 weeks that is guaranteed not to go moldy should therefore consider what they are getting into. Also, the crispy pretzels that are made in the bakery's oven from pale dough pieces can cause digestive disorders in sensitive individuals. In a conversation with the baker, he will surely be happy to explain the advantages of his baked goods, so that one can estimate what the differences between one bread and another are.

Upon closer examination of the current food horror, one would like to beam oneself back to the Stone Age and only eat roots, fruits, and insects.

Hardly anyone would really consider exchanging the comforts of civilization for times of hunger and cave bears. It makes more sense to explore the alternatives to industrially manufactured foods. How can one change one's diet sustainably so that it meets our biological needs? "Our needs", in this case, are the needs of the superorganism, i.e., the human being and the microbiome. To find this out, one should have the most important knowledge about the basic substances of our food. Therefore, you will find more information about what fills our plates and stomachs in the excursion "Macro and Micronutrients" in Chap. 8.

Dubious Ingredients: Emulsifiers, Sweeteners, Salt and Glyphosate

Many nutrition guides give the tip to cook meals yourself, instead of buying ready-made products and, especially, highly processed foods, a view that I strongly support. Not only because homemade dishes are probably healthier, but also because they are often cheaper, taste better and are more environmentally friendly due to less packaging waste. But before one condemns the chemistry in food across the board, one should know what one is talking about. Even though not all of the approximately 320 food additives allowed in Germany are harmful, there are a few substances that have gained dubious fame in the literature. Here are some prominent examples:

If you mix oil and vinegar for a salad dressing, the lighter oil rises to the surface after a short time, while the vinegar collects at the bottom. This separation is due to the different properties of fat and water. Similarly, in mayonnaise, margarine or ready-made soups, fat and water would separate from each other and the products would become lumpy if emulsifiers were not used. These substances link fat and water. They ensure that a product remains creamy, but also extend its shelf life or provide a pleasant consistency. Unconsciously, one uses such aids in the kitchen, for example, when making mayonnaise using egg yolk, which contains lecithin, among other things. Lecithin, alias E 322, is a food additive approved for food that is industrially obtained from rapeseed or soybeans. In addition to lecithin, the German additive approval regulation also lists about 40 other emulsifiers, some of which have fallen into disrepute.

One of the problematic emulsifiers is carboxymethyl cellulose (CMC), or E 466. For its production, fine cotton fibers are treated with the aggressive chemical trichloroacetic acid and can then bind water. CMC has no taste of its own and is not digested. The addition of E 466 to foods such as cream dishes, cream, fruit preparations, meat and fish products and baked goods prevents the separation of fat and water, increases the water holding capacity, and extends the shelf life. CMC is also used as a soluble fiber in low-calorie foods. The substance is considered unproblematic and there is no maximum quantity restriction.

Since emulsifiers have long been suspected of disturbing the intestinal barrier, the working group of the physician Prof. Alexander Swidsinki at the Charité in Berlin tested the effect of CMC on mice. A strain of animal that tends to have intestinal inflammation was used. Mice in the experimental group received CMC in their drinking water, while the control group drank pure water. After 3 weeks, it was found that bacteria had massively multiplied on the surface of the small intestine in the CMC animals. They filled the spaces between the intestinal villi, and the protective mucus layer was thinned. Inflammatory cells had migrated into the intestinal lumen: An intestinal inflammation had occurred (Swidsinski et al. 2009). A clear indication that emulsifiers like CMC, which are contained in many foods, could be partly responsible for intestinal inflammations in humans.

The topic was taken up by the working group of the biochemist Andrew Gewirtz at Georgia State University in Alabama and a much-noticed study appeared in the journal "Nature" in 2015. Gewirtz and his colleagues examined the effects of CMC and a second, also EU-approved emulsifier, polysorbate 80 (E 433), on different strains of mice, and found very similar effects as those discovered by Swidsinski (Chassaing et al. 2015). They found that the intestinal inflammation was due to damage to the intestinal barrier. Due to the emulsifiers, the mucus layer was thinner, so that bacteria could penetrate to the intestinal cells and irritate the immune system. The diversity of the intestinal flora had decreased in the emulsifier-treated animals and inflammation-promoting bacteria had spread. In addition, the mice in the experimental group ate more, gained more weight and had increased blood sugar levels, thus showing precursors of type 2 diabetes. The behavior of the mice was also changed by the emulsifier diet: among other things, the treated animals became less sociable (Holder et al. 2019). Interestingly, the chemical had no effect in mice that had no intestinal bacteria. So, bacteria played an important role in the disease process. This prompted further experiments and the scientists transferred intestinal bacteria from CMC mice to germ-free mice. In mice with such a bacterial transplantation, the known pathological changes occurred: accumulation of bacteria on the intestinal surface, thinning of mucus and inflammation. This conclusively proved that CMC alters the bacterial flora in mice and causes inflammation in this way.

It was alarming that the inflammatory effects were already apparent at very low doses of CMC in the drinking water or food of mice. The amounts of CMC corresponded to the concentrations of the substance found in many foods. This effect has since been confirmed in a carefully controlled study with 16 volunteers. The participants in the study consumed an amount of CMC with their food that is typical for a diet predominantly consisting of highly processed foods. In all individuals, CMC reduced the diversity of species in the gut and lowered the amount of anti-inflammatory metabolites, such as short-chain fatty acids. In some of the volunteers, the gut bacteria also penetrated deeply into the mucus layer of the intestine, promoting inflammation (Chassaing et al. 2021). It is clear that this food additive, which was considered harmless at the time of its approval in the 1960s when the microbiome was still an unknown entity, actually has massive, harmful effects.

Artificial sweeteners, often used to save calories, also affect the gut flora. A 3.3 g cube of sugar contains 13.5 kcal. To burn this energy, one would have to walk about 500 steps. For a 330 ml can of cola, which contains ten cubes of sugar, it would be 5000 steps. It is tempting to opt for the "Light" version instead of sugary products if you want to lose weight or maintain your current weight. Thus, artificial sweeteners have made a triumphant march around the world: Once only found in metallic-tasting diabetic drinks, they are now found in sodas and desserts of all kinds. However, those who use sugar substitutes hoping to stay slim or shed excess pounds may be in for a nasty surprise. Although overweight people often resort to sugar substitutes, experiments with mice show that synthetic sweeteners can have the opposite effect!

A much-cited study from the group led by Eran Elinav, Professor at the Weizmann Institute in Rehovot, Israel, showed that the legally permitted maximum amounts of the sugar substitutes aspartame, saccharin, and sucralose raised blood sugar levels in mice (Suez et al. 2014). Using saccharin as an example, the researchers went into detail and found that the sweetener turned the gut flora upside down. In mice that had been given saccharin, Bacteroides bacteria, which utilize food very efficiently, multiplied at the expense of other species. The blood sugar levels also increased as a result of the changed species composition of the gut flora. Such consistently high sugar levels lead to overweight and diabetes in the long run. The saccharin mice, indeed, had twice as much fat padding as their normally fed counterparts. When the researchers conducted the same experiment with mice without gut flora, the sugar levels remained normal. This made clear that, in the mice, it was not the sweetener itself, but the bacteria that drove up the blood sugar.

Does something similar also apply to humans? The Israeli group investigated this with seven volunteers who underwent a saccharin cure for a week.

They received saccharin three times a day, with a total amount that corresponded to the legally permitted maximum value. In studies with humans, one cannot expect numbers as clear as in a mouse experiment, because humans are not inbred, do not live under standard conditions, and have very individually different microbiomes. Nevertheless, four of the seven people reacted like the mice: Their gut flora changed and the blood sugar level increased. In three people, the values remained the same. When stool from the responding individuals was transferred to mice without gut flora, the bacteria contained therein increased the animals' blood sugar levels. The stool of non-responding individuals did not have this effect. The reaction of the microbiome to saccharin therefore seems to vary individually. However, anyone who has a microbiome that is susceptible to change by the artificial sweetener runs the risk of gaining weight instead of losing it! Eran Elinav has discussed the idea that artificial sweeteners may have contributed to the obesity epidemic they were originally developed to combat.

Also, additives that facilitate the processing of food or extend its shelf life can alter the gut flora or directly promote inflammation. Whether Phosphate in sausage to bind more water, maltodextrin as a fat substitute, problematic emulsifiers or artificial sweeteners: Many additives disrupt the balance of the gut flora, and thereby fuel inflammatory processes (Marion-Letellier et al. 2019). For example, carrageenan, a carbohydrate derived from algae that is also approved for organic foods according to European organic regulations, causes diarrhea, anemia, and weight loss in experimental animals. The effect of the thickening and gelling agent is based on changes in the gut microbiome (Shang et al. 2017; Naimi et al. 2021). The additives, which are usually not suspected in foods, are listed in long tables on 92 pages in the German Additive Approval Regulation. A total of 320 substances are listed there, ranging from substances such as beeswax and carob gum, which are considered harmless, to surfactants, which are also found in detergents and which you definitely do not want in your cake.

Even table salt, probably the oldest food additive and, at the same time, an essential mineral, has its pitfalls. In Germany, about 800 tons per day are sold, and an average person consumes about 7.5 g per day. This puts us well above the World Health Organization's recommended value of 5 g per day. Because the substance was always scarce, evolution has trained us to love salty food, which is why salt in ready-to-eat meals, sausages and snacks boosts sales. It has long been known that a salt-rich diet can lead to high blood pressure and heart disease. Thousands of studies prove this connection, but consumer behavior has not changed despite this.

That salt can also have an impact on inflammatory diseases was previously little known. An international group of researchers addressed this topic and examined the influence of our most important spice in mice. Food with increased salt content, as expected, drove up blood pressure and also promoted aggressive immune responses (Wilck et al. 2017). In mice with a disease similar to human multiple sclerosis, the salt-rich diet changed the species composition of the microbiome and intensified the disease symptoms. Particularly noticeable was a drastic decrease in lactobacilli, among which there are many probiotic strains. If lactobacilli were transplanted into mice that had become ill due to the salt diet, the inflammation values decreased and the disease symptoms were reduced, an indication of the role of the microbiome.

Volunteers in a study reacted similarly to the mice: If individuals were given an additional 4 g of table salt per day in addition to their normal food, their blood pressure and inflammation markers increased. At the same time, the number of lactobacilli decreased. The explanation: The lactobacilli, known to be sensitive, did not tolerate the increased salt content of the food and their populations shrank. These bacteria produce, among other things, the substance indole-3-lactic acid, which has a balancing effect on intestinal immune cells. Too much salt therefore leads to a reduced production of the calming molecule and promotes inflammation processes in this way: another reason to enjoy highly processed foods, which often contain a lot of salt, only with caution.

In addition to intentionally added food additives, which can be found in the register of the Federal Office for Nutrition, there are alarming traces of contaminants in probably every type of food. Books such as "Toxic Foods—the 10 deadliest poisons in our foods" (Wittwer 2017) draw attention to the health risk posed by pesticides, environmental toxins, plasticizers, and much more. Only rarely is the possible damage to the microbiome mentioned, although it is quite obvious. An example that illustrates this is glyphosate, the herbicide used worldwide that is now detectable everywhere in the eco-sphere. It inhibits an enzyme that is only found in plants and bacteria, but not in vertebrates, and thus has a far-reaching effect on all microbiomes (Van Bruggen et al. 2021). Of enormous importance is the fact that glyphosate also affects the microbiome of insects (Motta et al. 2018; Kiefer et al. 2021), and could thus contribute to the catastrophic insect die-off that threatens our entire eco-sphere (Milman 2022).

The toxicity of the substance was, as usual, demonstrated in animal experiments, in which the direct damage to mice was used as a benchmark. At the time of approval, no one thought of the microbiome.

However, it has since been found that glyphosate leads to shifts in the species composition in the microbiome of mice and rats, by pushing back useful commensal bacteria, such as lactobacilli, with harmful microbes (Tang et al. 2020). One consequence is an increased readiness for inflammation due to the loss of useful commensals. In addition, the herbicide kills bacteria that break down gluten, which could lead to an increased rate of celiac disease, according to corresponding articles (Barnett and Gibson 2020). It would be surprising if something similar did not also apply to the human microbiome. In this context, it is alarming that glyphosate is not only used to suppress weeds at the beginning of the vegetation period. Especially in North America, it is also sprayed again shortly before harvest because it accelerates the ripening of the grains. This also increases contamination. In Europe, people are more cautious, but European crops are also burdened. Despite the ubiquity of glyphosate and is very likely harmful effects, comprehensive, independent studies are rare as financial support for this kind of research is lacking. Although the proponents of a glyphosate ban put forward convincing arguments in intensive debates of the EU in 2023, the European Commission approved its continued use for another 10 years until 2034.

It would be too short-sighted to blame only the evil food industry for the increasing consumption of highly processed foods. After all, it responds to the wishes of consumers, who are, however, massively influenced by advertising and the design of the products. One of the most important reasons for buying highly processed foods, however, is low prices, as offered by discounters. Such low prices are only possible if products are made from cheap raw materials, which are often produced under unfair working conditions in countries of the global South, and that they are long-lasting, shape-stable and tasty through additives. These food additives are tested for their toxicity, but the main criteria in those tests were lethality and carcinogenicity in the mouse. At the time of approval of the substances, nothing was known about the microbiome and its possible effects. It is high time to review the list of food additives around this point and to set new limits for substances such as carboxy methyl cellulose or saccharin, or to ban them altogether. As long as this does not happen, one should avoid ready-made products at best and wield the cooking spoon whenever one can.

References

Baraldi LG et al (2018) Consumption of ultra-processed foods and associated sociodemographic factors in the USA between 2007 and 2012: evidence from a nationally representative cross-sectional study. BMJ Open 8:e020574

Barnett JA, Gibson DL (2020) Separating the empirical wheat from the pseudoscientific chaff: a critical review of the literature surrounding glyphosate, dysbiosis and wheat sensitivity. Front Microbiol 11:556729

Beslay M et al (2020) Ultra-processed food intake in association with BMI change and risk of overweight and obesity: a prospective analysis of the French NutriNet-Santé cohort. PLoS Med 17:e1003256

Chassaing B et al (2015) Dietary emulsifiers impact the mouse gut microbiota promoting colitis and metabolic syndrome. Nature 519:92–96

Chassaing B et al (2021) Randomized controlled feeding study of dietary emulsifier carboxymethylcellulose reveals detrimental impacts on the gut microbiota and metabolome. Gastroenterology 162:743–756

GBD 2017 Diet Collaborators (2019) Health effects of dietary risks in 195 countries, 1990–2017: a systematic analysis for the global burden of disease study 2017. Lancet 393:1958–1972

Geisslitz S et al (2019) Comparative study on gluten protein composition of ancient (einkorn, emmer and spelt) and modern wheat species (durum and common wheat). Food Secur 8:409

Ho JY, Hendi AS (2018) Recent trends in life expectancy across high income countries: retrospective observational study. BMJ 362:K2562

Hoch T et al (2013) Manganese-enhanced magnetic resonance imaging for mapping of whole brain activity patterns associated with the intake of snack food in ad libitum fed rats. PLoS One 8:e55354

Hoch T et al (2015) Fat/carbohydrate ratio but not energy density determines snack food intake and activates brain reward areas. Sci Rep 14:10041

Holder MK et al (2019) Dietary emulsifier consumption alters anxiety-like and social-related behaviors in mice in a sex-dependent manner. Sci Rep 9:172

Juul F et al (2015) Trends in consumption of ultra-processed foods and obesity in Sweden between 1960 and 2010. Publ Health Nutr 18:3091–3107

Kiefer JST et al (2021) Inhibition of a nutritional endosymbiont by glyphosate abolishes mutualistic benefit on cuticle synthesis in Oryzae-philus surinamensis. Commun Biol 4:554

Kiehnle H (1927) Kindle Kochbuch: Große Illustrierte Ausgabe für die bürgerliche und feine Küche. Tausend, Süddeutsches Verlagshaus GmbH, Stuttgart, pp 49–53

Longin CFH et al (2020) Influence of wheat variety and dough preparation on FODMAP content in yeast-leavened wheat breads. J Cereal Sci 95:103021

Marion-Letellier R et al (2019) Inflammatory bowel diseases and food additives: to add fuel on the flames! Nutrients 11:1111

Milman O (2022) The insect crisis: the fall of the tiny empires that rule the world. Atlantic Books, London

Motta EVS et al (2018) Glyphosate perturbs the gut microbiota of honey bees. PNAS 115:10305–10310

Naimi S et al (2021) Direct impact of commonly used dietary emulsifiers on human gut microbiota. Microbiome 9:66

RKI (2014). https://www.rki.de/DE/Content/Gesundheitsmonitoring/Themen/Uebergewicht_Adipositas/Uebergewicht_Adipositas_node.html.   Accessed 3 July 2020

Santos-Costa C et al (2017) Consumption of ultra-processed foods and body fat during childhood and adolescence: a systematic review. Publ Health Nutr 21:148–159

Schnabel L et al (2019) Association between ultraprocessed food consumption and risk of mortality among middle-aged adults in France. JAMA Intern Med 179:490–498

Schuppan D, Gisbert-Schuppan K (2018) Tägliches Brot: Krank durch Weizen, Gluten and ATI. Springer-Verlag GmbH

Shang Q et al (2017) Carrageenan-induced colitis is associated with decreased population of the anti-inflammatory bacterium, Akkermansia muciniphila, in the gut microbiota of C57BL/6J mice. Toxicol Lett 279:87–95

Suez J et al (2014) Artificial sweeteners induce glucose intolerance by altering the gut microbiota. Nature 514:181–186

Swidsinski A et al (2009) Bacterial overgrowth and inflammation of small intestine after carboxymethylcellulose ingestion in genetically susceptible mice. Inflamm Bowel Dis 15:359–364

Tang Q et al (2020) Glyphosate exposure induces inflammatory responses in the small intestine and alters gut microbial composition in rats. Environ Pollut 261:114129

Van Bruggen AHC et al (2021) Indirect effects of the herbicide glyphosate on plant, animal and human health through its effects on microbial communities. Front Environ Sci 617:255–268

WHO (2017). https://www.who.int/news/item/11-10-2017-tenfold-increase-in-childhood-and-adolescent-obesity-in-four-decades-new-study-by-imperial-college-london-and-who. Accessed 3 Mar 2022

Wilck N et al (2017) Salt-responsive gut commensal modulates TH17 axis and disease. Nature 551:585–589

Wittwer P (2017) Giftige Lebensmittel – die 10 tödlichsten Gifte in unseren Lebensmitteln. Amazon.de: Kindle-Shop

Ziegler JU et al (2016) Wheat and the irritable bowel syndrome– FODMAP levels of modern and ancient species and their retention during bread making. J Funct Foods 25:257–266

Zinöcker MK, Lindseth IA (2018) The western diet-microbiome-host interaction and its role in metabolic disease. Nutrients 10:365

7

More Attention for Our Inner Ecosystem!

Contents

A New Pact with Our Inhabitants

It took decades for science to take note of the alarming increase in inflammatory diseases and to intensively investigate the causes. Initially, it was believed that the decline in infections was responsible for the sharp increase in cases of disease ("hygiene hypothesis"), after which the importance of environmental bacteria as an inflammation brake ("farm effect") was recognized. Today, the anti-inflammatory effect of the microbiome is the focus of attention. These three explanations for the increase in inflammatory diseases do not contradict each other; on the contrary, they complement each other: All agree that, without certain, dampening signals from bacteria, the human immune system is misprogrammed, runs too high and tends towards inflammation.

Those who are lucky enough to have grown up on an organic farm with a rich bacterial flora and continue to live there should best skip the following pages. He or she would probably have a very diverse microbiome and a relatively tolerant immune system that ignores irrelevant stimuli. The probability of inflammatory diseases would be similarly low as in indigenous peoples. The many others, however, who, like almost every person in an industrialized country, have adopted the Western lifestyle, should think about the cohabitation with their commensals. Homo sapiens is no longer exposed to the microbes that our immune system needs to function optimally. This lack is most clearly evident in the microbiome: Compared to people living close to nature, the inner ecosystem of the modern city dweller is poor in bacterial species and the existing inhabitants brake immune responses less efficiently. The result is an increased risk of the modern human for inflammatory diseases such as allergies, autoimmune diseases and food intolerances.

In modern societies, almost all people have a disturbed relationship with their 40 trillion inhabitants. We have maltreated our inner shared living space, much like we have brought our outer living world to the brink of collapse. Modern nutrition, improperly applied medications, lack of exercise and too little contact with nature have caused a decline in the species diversity of our inhabitants. The inner ecosystem is dominated by species that led a niche existence in our ancestors, while other species that used to calm the immune system with their products have disappeared from the scene. This imbalance must be turned upside down again. We need a new pact with our commensals, we must give them back the space they need to keep us healthy!

How can one, without beaming back to the Middle Ages, achieve the necessary bacterial diversity, and thus favorably influence the immune system? The most effective way is to create the right conditions early in childhood. Playing outdoors, contact with soil, animals and dirt and early acclimatization to diverse food, instead of an overprotected existence in a sterile bubble, would be an important start. But what if one has already left childhood behind, grew up in a germ-poor city apartment and fully enjoyed the Western lifestyle? Can the possibly misprogrammed immune system then be reprogrammed?

There is no "reset" button that one can press, but the answer is still "Yes!"—because epidemiological studies show that good nutrition, healthy lifestyle and a diverse microbial environment prevent inflammatory diseases. This correlation can also be traced in mouse models; for example, the onset of type 1 diabetes can be prevented by a suitable diet (Marino et al. 2017). A similar language is also spoken by current studies on COVID-19 infections in humans, where a clear connection exists between anti-inflammatory microbiome and less severe courses of the disease (Zuo et al. 2020).

But can a change in the internal and external microbial diversity also improve the course of an existing inflammatory disease? Nutritional studies, in which groups of subjects consumed different diets over certain periods of time, suggest this. Such intervention studies show that diets with a high proportion of plant-based foods have a positive effect on autoimmune diseases (Wagenaar et al. 2021). In mice, existing type 1 diabetes diseases can be alleviated with suitable food that optimizes the microbiome (Marino et al. 2017), and diseases similar to asthma can also be significantly improved (Thorburn et al. 2015). Similar effects are also seen with environmental bacteria or exercise.

Everything therefore suggests that a disturbed balance with the commensals can be improved by changing the lifestyle. But which way is the most efficient? Where should the focus be placed?

In addition to healthy eating, i.e., preferably natural food with a high proportion of plants and lots of dietary fiber, one can consciously incorporate plenty of exercise, pets and contact with soil into family life. A dip in the bathing lake (instead of in sterile chlorinated swimming pool water) can also help to enrich the microbiome with new species. In cases in which a previous illness or treatment with antibiotics have stressed the microbiome, probiotics or even a stool transplant can help, as will be discussed further below.

However, these measures are not comparable in their mode of action to a pill that you swallow and a short time later the toothache is gone. Because our microbes approach their tasks in a division of labor, a balanced equilibrium of species has usually been established in the intestine, on the skin, and on the mucous membranes that reacts to changes in the short term, but usually swings back to the basic state in the long term. In the healthy intestine, our 40 trillion inhabitants have settled in with each other and staked out their territories. Through a strategy of occupied chairs, which also keeps disease-causing germs at bay, they keep new bacteria, which represent competition, under control. Only through long-lasting changes do the balances among the species shift, with new bacteria also getting a chance to establish themselves. A different diet, gardening, or a dog improve contact with bacteria only if they become part of everyday life. A change in the microbiome will therefore only work if lifestyle habits are also permanently changed, without reverting to old patterns. It is therefore important to invest time and to have patience. But what could be more tempting than securing your health with such simple means as healthy eating, exercise, and contact with nature, while giving your commensals the attention they need?

Better Nutrition

Healthy eating is one of the best investments in your own future. What sounds like a truism is scientifically well proven. The highest-ranking statement on this comes from the EAT-Lancet Commission, a highly respected international panel of experts, in which 37 scientists from various fields from 16 countries work together. In 2019, this commission calculated that unhealthy eating poses a higher health risk than smoking, alcohol, unprotected sex, and drugs combined (Willet et al. 2019). Those who eat healthily have a significantly higher life expectancy. Better nutrition is therefore recommended to everyone! Details on nutrition can be found in the "Micro- and Macronutrients" section in Chap. 8.

But what kind of "healthy eating" works best against inflammation? If you stand in a large bookstore in front of the health and nutrition section, the diversity can be quite overwhelming. The spectrum of diets ranges from low carb to high protein, and from Ayurvedic to Mediterranean. And all promise health, well-being, and even, in some cases, a dream figure.

So, let's ask science: Experts agree that we should consume fewer unhealthy saturated fats, fewer calories, and more plant-based dietary fiber. This type of diet reduces the risk of inflammatory diseases, but also of other lifestyle diseases. The positive effect of plant-based food is supported by many studies. The most famous study from which we draw nutritional data on this topic is the Nurses' Health Study from the USA. It started in 1976, and currently includes about 280,000 participants. Nurses, who diligently document their patients' data every day, are readily trusted to also keep a record of their own health behavior. To investigate the influence of diet on chronic inflammatory bowel diseases such as Crohn's disease and ulcerative colitis, the collected data was sorted according to dietary behavior, and groups of people who either predominantly ate plant-based or had a high proportion of animal products in their diet were formed. For example, it was found that, with a fiber-rich, predominantly plant-based diet, the risk of chronic inflammatory bowel diseases was less than half as high as with a diet low in fiber (Ananthakrishnan et al. 2013).

Studies with volunteers suggest what experiments with mice have shown some time ago, namely, that the positive effect of plant fibers is due to the microbiome (Menni et al. 2021; Asnicar et al. 2021). Plant substances that can only be broken down by bacteria in the large intestine provide gut bacteria with the food they need to produce positively acting metabolic products such as short-chain fatty acids, but also other anti-inflammatory metabolites. Accordingly, most dietary studies, in which large amounts of fiber are used, lead to an increase in bacteria such as Faecalibacterium, Eubacterium or Roseburia, which produce short-chain fatty acids. Parallel to the increase in beneficial bacteria, most studies show a decrease in inflammatory markers in the blood, and sometimes also an improvement in the clinical picture of inflammatory diseases (Wagenaar et al. 2021).

A complete cure of inflammatory diseases through a change in diet is not evident from the published studies. However, this does not rule out that a cure can be achieved in individual cases.

So, by designing one's menu, one has an important key to an anti-inflammatory microbiome that prevents inflammatory diseases. The question arises as to how much fiber is needed to really overhaul one's microbiome. A meta-study, in which 30 dietary studies are analyzed, speaks clearly: Eating just a little more fruit or vegetables every day does not have a sufficient effect. Anyone who wants to change their microbiome must be willing to incorporate large amounts of fiber into their diet plan or should ideally switch to a vegetarian or vegan lifestyle (Wagenaar et al. 2021). Remember, African hunters and gatherers, who rarely suffer from inflammatory diseases, consume more than 100 g of fiber daily. The German Society for Nutrition recommends 30 g of fiber as a minimum, but, on average, only 20 g per person is achieved. Therefore, meals should generally contain much more dietary fibers than before. So: Whole grain products and vegetables, vegetables, vegetables on the table!

Plant fibers are important for another reason: A frequently overlooked consequence of the Western lifestyle is the loss of species in the microbiome. Let's remember that hunters and gatherers have about 60% more species of gut bacteria than healthy, modern living humans. In people with inflammatory diseases, this species diversity is often even further reduced. However, the diversity of gut bacteria ensures the stability of the system against disturbances. Anyone who wants to replenish their depleted microbiome through healthy nutrition should ensure not only a sufficient quantity, but also a great diversity of dietary fibers and secondary plant substances.

Not without reason does the German Society for Nutrition recommend at least five portions of different fruits or vegetables a day. Ideally, this plant-based freshness cure should also be as colorful and vibrant as possible, because with blue, red and yellow plant substances, a wide spectrum of important secondary plant substances is covered. In this sense, a recommendation from Tim Spector, a guru of the British nutrition scene, is: "Eat the rainbow"— because those who eat colorfully live healthily. Such a plant-focused diet supports an anti-inflammatory microbiome, whose bacteria are good producers of short-chain fatty acids and other positive metabolites. On the other hand, those who frequently have highly processed foods and animal products on the menu breed Proteobacteria, with their inflammation-promoting bacterial danger signals and unfavorable Firmicutes such as Ruminococcus and Blautia (Bolte et al. 2021).

Anyone who wants to make their diet healthier will also hardly be able to avoid reducing their sugar consumption, which is absorbed by the small intestine and leaves the microbiome in the large intestine starving. By avoiding sweets, you also avoid many industrial foods to which sugar has been added to improve the taste. With their emulsifiers, preservatives, trans fats and other additives, they stress the microbiome. Similarly, by avoiding sugary soft drinks and sweets, you also avoid calories that lead to inflammation-promoting overweight (see below). It is amazing how little effort it takes to reduce sugar consumption. Sweet food and sweet drinks are purely a matter of habit!

But it's not only sugar itself: starch-based foods that release sugar in the intestine in the short term should also be reduced. It is now known that our commensal bacteria do not benefit from white flour products like white bread or pasta. The fact that potatoes and rice also mainly consist of easily degradable starch, which is unfavorable for the microbiome, has hardly been spread. However, if you choose the whole grain version for grain products, you are already better off in terms of health, as the nutrients are harder to access, so that a part benefits the commensals in the large intestine. The same applies to potatoes, rice and pasta, if you let them cool down after cooking and use them afterwards. When cooling down, part of the starch condenses and can no longer be broken down by the enzymes of the small intestine, but is good food for the bacteria in the large intestine.

The emphasis on plant-based nutrition indirectly means a reduction in the proportion of meat in the diet. In fact, it is clear that such a change promotes health and increases life expectancy. A large meta-study by the WHO (IARC 2018) is groundbreaking in this respect. Here, processed meat products were classified in the highest stage of carcinogenic substances, and red meat (beef, pork, mutton, etc.) was classified as potentially carcinogenic (see also the excursion "Macro and micronutrients" in Chap. 8). In addition, red meat also promotes bacteria that produce the harmful trimethylamine, which is converted into TMAO in the liver, leading to heart diseases. Accordingly, The German Society for Nutrition recommends a reduction in meat consumption from the current average of about 1100 g to a maximum of 600 g per person per week (DGE 2021). The previously mentioned EAT-Lancet study (Willet et al. 2019) goes even further with its recommendations, and calls for a reduction in meat consumption to 300 g per week for the sake of health and sustainability. This is equivalent to about one thin slice of ham per day. Such a switch from animal to plant-based foods also promotes the health of the planet. After all, animal proteins have a carbon footprint several times higher than plant proteins. While the production of 100 g of lentil protein generates

250 g of CO2, the production of 100 g of protein from pork requires almost eight times that amount, namely, 1939 g of CO2!

What else should be considered when trying to make one's diet microbiome-friendly? Experienced nutritionists often emphasize how difficult it is to maintain dietary changes. But, since long-term change is the goal, it's best to take into account one's own preferences when experimenting. If you absolutely don't like spinach, you shouldn't frustrate yourself with this vegetable! It's best to pick out the components from various suggestions that appeal to you the most. If you consider four points when putting together your diet, you're already on the right track:

- High proportion of plant-based dietary fiber.
- Low sugar and starch-based foods, healthy fats.
- High variety of food.
- Cook yourself, avoiding highly processed foods with their harmful additives.

A good choice for me would be a versatile, mainly plant-based diet like the Mediterranean diet. This diet provides the gut flora with plenty of plant fibers thanks to vegetables and legumes, while olive oil provides valuable unsaturated fatty acids, seafood contributes omega-3 fatty acids, and a moderate proportion of animal foods rounds out the protein supply. Instead of meeting the need for omega-3 fatty acids through fish, flaxseed oil, rapeseed oil, or microalgae can also be sources. Berries and fruit provide important secondary plant substances, such as polyphenols. In northern latitudes, which includes Central Europe, an additional vitamin D supply is advisable, as the UV radiation is not sufficient to provide modern humans with adequate amounts. Moderation in terms of calories and regular physical activity are also important.

With a similar diet, the inhabitants of the "Blue Zones" mentioned in the second chapter reach an above-average old age in good health. This type of diet corresponds quite well to human physiology, as we are designed as omnivores, with a gut whose length lies between that of herbivores and carnivores. Viewed through the lens of evolution, we and our microbiome live best with a corresponding mixed diet, as we have adapted to a life as hunters and gatherers over millions of years.

However, when changing your diet, you should also consider that an anti-inflammatory microbiome is not a magic bullet that guarantees slimness at the same time. Certainly, avoiding calorie-dense foods with a high proportion of starch, sugar, and unfavorable fats is an important step towards weight reduction. But even an excess of healthy foods can lead to fat deposits, whose fat cells incessantly produce inflammation-promoting adipokines. These calorie stores are even partly filled by the "good", anti-inflammatory bacteria that break down plant dietary fibers, and thereby produce calming short-chain fatty acids. These molecules are not only anti-inflammatory, because they support regulatory T cells, but also provide calories at the same time. If you want to strengthen your immune tolerance, you also have to pay attention to your body weight and live a healthy lifestyle all around. In any case, such a comprehensive change will be a long-lasting process that must be done step by step.

More Exercise

Sport and exercise do not only strengthen the muscles and the circulation, counteract obesity and improve metabolism. Regular exercise also lowers inflammation markers and has positive effects on autoimmune diseases. Physically active individuals have a lower risk of developing rheumatoid arthritis, multiple sclerosis, chronic intestinal inflammation or psoriasis, and the course of the diseases is milder than in comparatively inactive persons (Sharif et al. 2018). These effects are attributed to a changed balance in the immune system. On the one hand, the anti-inflammatory messenger substances released by muscles during activation, the myokines, play an important role. They are also involved in the breakdown of storage fat. On the other hand, exercise also directly affects the microbiome, which, in turn, has an anti-inflammatory effect. Comparisons between active people and couch potatoes showed an increase in regulatory T cells, which suppress inflammation processes, in athletes. Even when individuals engaged in intensive sports for 3 hours per week, potentially anti-inflammatory bacterial species such as Faecalibacterium prausnizii, Roseburia hominis and Akkermansia muciniphila increased (Mailing 2019).

How exercise changes the microbiome and how the bacteria then affect the human immune system is not fully understood. Interesting clues, however, come from studies in rodents. Here, a several-week exercise training of the animals favors bacterial species that produce short-chain fatty acids from plant fibers (Matsumoto et al. 2008). As shown earlier, these small molecules provide energy and simultaneously shift the balance of T cells towards regulatory T cells. So, it is not surprising that animals that get little exercise are more likely to develop intestinal inflammation than mice trained on a running wheel (Cook et al. 2016). Transfer experiments showed that the positive effect of physical activity can be transferred with the microbiome, similar to the effect on the fat- or slimming effect of the microbiome. When the gut bacteria of trained mice were transplanted to germ-free animals, the recipients were protected from intestinal inflammations, while the control animals fell ill (Allen et al. 2017).

Exercise also reduces inflammation in another way: Those who move a lot store less fat. In particular, the dangerous the abdominal fat inside the abdominal cavity that produces inflammatory messengers. These adipokines contribute to the risk of many inflammatory diseases. Thus, in the previously mentioned Nurses' Health Study, the risk of chronic intestinal inflammation in overweight individuals was twice as high as in normal-weight individuals (Harper and Zisman 2016). An excess of pounds has also been described as a risk factor for multiple sclerosis, asthma, type 1 diabetes, rheumatoid arthritis and other inflammatory diseases. So, if you avoid overweight, either by reduced calorie intake or increased energy expenditure through exercise, you live more healthily. Those who maintain their slim figure through physical activity do even more for their health due to the multitude of positive effects of exercise than the mere calorie cutter.

How you get exercise and what kind of sport you engage in is less important. Sports medicine specialists advise people to just get moving and not to set goals that are too high, because excessive ambition often leads to the cessation of activities, and thus to a relapse into old habits. For example, if one manages to walk an additional 2000 steps on top of the usual distance covered per day, much is already gained. Outdoor exercise is particularly healthy, as it also replenishes one's vitamin D stores.

More Contact with Nature

Another important factor that determines our microbiome and the immune response is contact with nature in the broadest sense. As mentioned earlier, a decrease in diversity of microbial species in the environment reduces the tendency towards inflammatory diseases. Whether the bacteria come from animals, cow barn dust, untreated water, forest soil or garden soil certainly makes a difference, but the details as to why are not known. The mechanisms are also unclear: Do, for example, the bacteria that mediate the healing effect of traditional farms act through the skin or the lungs, or are they incorporated into the microbiome of the gut? And, if so, do they become a permanent part of the gut flora or are they just short-term visitors? Here, too, the data is still sparse. But one thing is clear: A relatively primal life with a lot of contact with nature supports the anti-inflammatory mechanisms of the immune system. The comparisons presented earlier between the lifestyles of children in the

Finnish and Russian parts of Karelia, with their very different disease frequencies, fit into this pattern (see Chap. 2 "How our life has changed has"). The aspect of contact with nature has been particularly emphasized in the Finnish scientific scene. No wonder that this topic is being intensively worked on there, because, on the one hand, Finland is one of the most forest-rich countries in the world and prides itself on having the cleanest air, but, on the other hand, the Finns hold world records in terms of inflammatory diseases. The Finns love nature and attribute healing effects to it. However, more than 90% of the inhabitants of the country do not live in the forest or by a lake, but rather lead a modern, urban life. In the cities, the sealing of the surfaces with concrete and asphalt is well advanced and, for reasons of hygiene, schoolyards and the outdoor areas of kindergartens are also concreted.

Such impoverishment of the environment has consequences: Children who have little contact with nature suffer more frequently from inflammatory diseases. In one study, the environment of the homes of both allergic and healthy children was analyzed for the spectrum of plant species within a radius of three kilometers. Allergic children demonstrably lived in a less diverse environment than their healthy peers. Healthy children had more access to forests and agricultural areas—and thus to a richer flora and fauna, with the corresponding microbes. As a result, the healthy children had a more diverse skin microbiome (Hanski et al. 2012).

This raises the question of whether more nature in daily life can break the trend towards ever more inflammatory diseases, in short, whether nature can act as a medicine. The ecologist Prof. Aki Sinkkonen from the University of Helsinki wondered what would happen if nature were to be brought back into a microbially impoverished environment, and started a simple experiment to determine the answer. Sinkkonen equipped the sealed play areas of conventional kindergartens with forest soil, turf sods, planting beds and peat blocks for playing and romping. Unchanged, conventional kindergartens served as a control. It was ensured that the children spent about 1.5 hours per day outside and engaged with the introduced material. Before the changes and 28 days later, at the end of the experiment, the microbiome of the skin, the composition of the gut flora and inflammatory values in the blood were analyzed. The results were clear. Even in this relatively short period of time, contact with natural material had increased the diversity of skin bacteria and changed the gut flora of the children. Even more impressive, however, was that inflammatory values in the blood had decreased and the number of regulatory T cells had increased in the experimental group (Roslund et al. 2020). The increased contact with nature had obviously strengthened the children's immune tolerance!

My question as to whether contact with soil could also pose a risk of pathogens was answered very clearly by Aki Sinkkonen in a telephone interview: In temperate climates, one need not particularly fear pathogens; a tetanus vaccination is important, but other pathogens play no major role. The soil bacteria are essentially harmless, but he would assume that they stimulate the immune system similarly to related pathogens, and thus slow down inflammatory responses with repeated contact (see also Chap. 4 on the microbiome).

If one researches which environmental bacteria could be associated with tolerance, one repeatedly comes across gamma-proteobacteria (Hanski et al. 2012; Fyhrquist et al. 2014; Ruokolainen et al. 2025), which belong to the gram-negative bacteria, whose surface components are pro-inflammatory. In particular, the genus Acinetobacter should be focused upon. These germs are usually met with suspicion: The Acinetobacter species is quite resistant to external influences and is found in soil, water, dust and on plants, but also on the skin and in the respiratory tract of healthy individuals. Usually, the bacteria behave peacefully, but in individuals with a weakened immune system, they can become opportunistic pathogens. If the immune system does not keep them in check, they spread and can lead to pneumonia or purulent inflammations in various organs. Acinetobacter can, in rare cases, even enter the bloodstream, and thus cause deadly sepsis.

So, are environmental bacteria like Acinetobacter crucial for immune tolerance? In an interview, immunologist Prof. Harri Alenius from the University of Helsinki explained to me that the Finns do not doubt the role of the gut flora, and thus the importance of diet, but, in addition, they believe that the environmental bacteria are also an important factor. He explains that, in Finland, there are large differences in disease frequency between urban and rural areas. However, the food supply in supermarkets would not differ at all between Helsinki and a remote small town, and the eating habits of the population are largely the same. However, the bacterial landscape in the people's environments is different. Therefore, the gamma-proteobacteria are considered as a cause for the lower frequency of inflammatory diseases in rural areas. Interestingly, these bacteria have the potential to influence the immune system, as some colonize the skin (Naktsuji et al. 2013; Bay et al. 2020) or stimulate mucosal cells of the lung. It is not clear whether Acinetobacter is the decisive bacterium or whether other bacteria that occur with it are more important.

A component of the complex surface of the gamma-proteobacteria is the LPS described in the microbiome chapter, which puts the innate immune system on alert even in the smallest concentrations. In the long term, however, contact with LPS contributes to tolerance (see the section "Microbial

Danger Signals" in Chap. 4). Especially in the phase that shapes the immune system, early childhood, this programming is anchored through epigenetic changes. The immune system—per Alenius—needs such bacterial stimuli from the natural environment of humans for the development of immune tolerance. With this view, the Finnish researchers are in good company, as the gamma-proteobacteria are also at the top of the list of potentially immune-modulating bacteria in studies on the farm effect (see Chap. 3) (Debarry et al. 2007).

Are there, therefore, other important factors at play in addition to diet that influence the tendency towards inflammation? Does contact with nature perhaps have an even greater significance? In-depth studies that make a clear statement on this matter are rare. A very impressive work comes from the team around Fergus Shanahan from the University of Cork in Ireland (Keohane et al. 2010). The authors examined the lifestyle and microbiomes of the travelling people in Ireland, the "Irish Travellers". To understand this, some background is needed: The Travellers make up about 1% of the Irish population and used to live nomadically as horse traders, farm workers, tin-smiths, and entertainers. Genetically, they are close to the Irish, so they are not, for example, Sinti or Roma. Around the turn of the millennium, the Irish government intensified its efforts to settle this ethnic group, forcing many Travellers to live in fixed dwellings. Thus, among the Travellers today, there are various stages of sedentary life or free life as travelling people.

The disappearing world of the nomadic Travellers is captured in an article in National Geographic from 2016. The images impressively show how large families with an average of 9.8 children (compared to 1.38 children in the Irish population) live in caravans at changing locations. A large part of their time is spent outdoors and in contact with horses, dogs, and other people. Television and computer games seem to play no role. With increasing seden-tary life, this picture changes: People live in simple, dreary dwellings on the outskirts of cities. They have more access to sanitary facilities and medical care but spend much less time outdoors. The microbiomes of the people reflect this transition in lifestyle: The microbiomes of the still nomadic Travellers show similarities with those of hunters and gatherers, but with a more seden-tary life, they increasingly resemble the "western microbiomes" of the Irish population.

What does not differ between nomadic and sedentary Travellers is their diet! Both groups eat similarly unhealthily, with a high proportion of animal proteins and fat and low amounts of dietary fibre. Nevertheless, inflammatory diseases are only slightly present among the Travellers; for example, chronic intestinal inflammations are virtually unknown. The scientists identified the type of housing, the number of children in the family, and the keeping of animals as factors that make a difference between the Travellers and the Irish population, using complex statistical methods. All these factors cause a constant exchange of bacteria with the environment, with these bacteria then also becoming part of the microbiome. The take-home message: Close cohabitation with other people and animals under conditions that favor exchange of bacteria creates a balanced microbiome and reduces the likelihood of inflammatory diseases. The data from the Traveller study thus support the Finnish assessment of the importance of environmental bacteria and also confirm the hygiene hypothesis and the farm effect.

If one reads health studies with a sharpened view, there are also indications in other works that the Fergus Shanahan group is not alone in its findings. For example, a study of immigrants from a Thai mountain tribe in the USA found that their microbiome became less diverse the longer they stayed in the host country (Vangay et al. 2018). This finding is not surprising. What distinguishes the study, however, is the simultaneous examination of eating behaviour. Here, the authors find—somewhat surprisingly, one might think—that eating behaviour does not differ between the first and second generation of immigrants. The children of the immigrated Asians continue to eat the traditional diet, but have a "western" microbiome. The authors calculate using complex statistical methods that, in this case, diet has only a minor influence on the composition of the microbiome. Which factors are decisive remains open, but it is quite conceivable that the microbiome thinned out because the immigrants were no longer exposed to the bacterial diversity of their native villages, but instead lived in a biologically impoverished environment on the outskirts of American cities. It is to be hoped that this relationship between environment and microbiome, as well as the resulting disease risks, will be much more strongly focused on than before.

Inspirations from the New Health Scene

The Western lifestyle, despite its inflammatory diseases and the obesity epidemic with its far-reaching negative consequences, is rarely seriously questioned, but continues to stand for prosperity and quality of life. Even well-informed health enthusiasts often find a fundamental change in lifestyle habits too cumbersome, because, after all, they have survived quite well so far. Why then make additional efforts? It's easier to paint reality in rosy colors.

Let's take nutrition as an example: In the annual representative Forsa survey of the Federal Ministry of Agriculture in 2021, 84% of 1000 consumers stated that they eat healthily. 76% of respondents said they eat vegetables and fruit daily and 52% said they cook almost daily. For the nutritionist Prof. Hans Hauner from the Technical University of Munich, this result does not match data from nutrition studies. Investigations that specifically measure the consumption of test persons show that a clear majority of the subjects consume less than the recommended amount of vegetables and fruit, and more than half of their carbohydrates come in the form of sugar. The amount of dietary fiber, on the other hand, is much too low. In addition, the consumption of highly processed, energy-dense, and therefore unhealthy, foods is constantly increasing. As a result, the average citizen's diet is anything but healthy. It is too fatty and too calorie-rich, and therefore not very health-promoting. This, according to Prof. Hauner, explains why about half of the women and two-thirds of the men in Germany are overweight.

Obviously, the statements of the surveyed consumers reflect their good intention to eat healthily. Unfortunately, many of these good projects are then not implemented due to convenience, financial reasons or lack of time, and people resort to convenience products, instead of treating themselves to a healthy meal. A look at the food offerings at gas stations, where especially young people get their evening meal, speaks volumes.

A very similar discrepancy exists in relation to exercise: The good intention to go for a walk, a jog or a visit to the soccer field is there, but when it gets concrete, the lure of media is too tempting, and people end up spending all of their time in front of the screen. As a result, people in modern societies have never engaged in as little movement as they do today, a fact that is especially true for children and adolescents.

However, there are also many people who behave more consciously. A growing proportion of the population is actively engaging with health today, and older people are especially aware that health is not a given. Healthy nutrition, as well as physical and mental fitness, is in the foreground. According to a survey by the Allensbach Institute, in 2021, 7.5 million people in Germany described themselves as vegetarians (9%) and 1.13 million (1.5%) as vegans. This proportion has been steadily increasing over the past few years. Big cities like Berlin are a kind of future lab, where upcoming developments become visible early on. One good indicator that I see for changes in diet is the existence of organic supermarkets. Organic food is experiencing a real boom, in Germany, their turnover has more than doubled from 2010 to 2020, and now accounts for over 6% of the market volume. In Berlin, branches of BioCompany, Dennree, Alnatura and LPG are springing up in every neighborhood like mushrooms. When shopping, I always wonder how much money people, especially young people, who usually do not have a lavish income, invest in high-quality food.

When you talk to bio-affine customers and ask them why they do what they do, it turns out that most of them think about health, animal welfare, and climate together. They want to live healthily, eat good-tasting food, and, at the same time, do something for the farm animals and rescue the over-heated planet. They also like to buy regionally to avoid long transport routes, with their large CO2 footprint, and to support the local (agricultural) economy. The climate balance is also taken into account when choosing food: less meat, but of better quality, and from sustainable production of humanely kept animals is very much in trend. After all, the rearing, slaughtering, and processing of one kilogram of poultry or pork produces 4.3 times the amount of CO2 as the production of one kilo of mixed bread. With beef, it's even 18 times the amount! Therefore, a more plant-based diet, which saves CO2 and requires less water and land for cultivation, is much more sustainable.

The public sector, with its canteens, kindergartens, and schools, is only hesitantly implementing these findings. Some major cities have developed nutritional guidelines in cooperation with interest groups and consumer organizations. For example, in Munich, it was decided that 10% of the products used in the city's canteens must be organic, while, in kindergartens, this share is 50%, and for meat, even as high as 100%. There are also specific requirements for regional and seasonal products. However, some organizations go beyond such guidelines on their own initiative. The menu of the Berlin university canteens is now largely vegetarian. After student representatives advocated for a "canteen revolution", the conventional canteens began to offer a meat-containing meal on only 2 days, in addition to several vegetarian dishes, and on Fridays, a meal with fish is on the menu. What's more, there is a completely vegetarian canteen, and even a "deep green" vegan canteen (Ernährungsrat Berlin 2021). These are at least steps towards a healthy diet, but one should keep in mind that "organic" alone does not guarantee health. Even if sugar is made from 100% organically grown sugar beets, it is still sugar. And a diet that consists mainly of rice pudding and pasta is not healthy, even if it is vegetarian.

When asked why this alternative, more plant-based diet is healthier, the argument often comes up that the food is "lighter" and "less burdensome". People have heard of bacteria in the gut, but they are rarely associated with health. However, it is obvious that the effects of nutrition are largely determined by the microbiome. But only a hard core of health-conscious people have this connection on their radar and also think about optimizing the microbiome.

Many of the health-conscious people I talk to have a pronounced antenna for fitness and sports. Before the Corona pandemic, membership in a gym was more the rule than the exception. Many of the respondents trained two to three times a week on cardio machines or did strength training, or they attended aerobic or fitness classes. The Corona pandemic has interrupted this routine, but, in the meantime, many of them have switched to jogging, cycling, or making sure they get enough exercise by consulting the pedometer on their smartphones every day. Fitness bracelets and watches are also very popular. With an Apple Watch on your arm, a device that not only tells the time, but also transmits biometric data and allows for phone calls and internet access, you can document your commitment. All these devices are useful if they help to overcome the inner laziness that ties you to the screen. It makes you proud to be in good shape and to be efficient. A lot of energy is invested in this, and this effort pays off in everyday life, both professionally and privately. However, the connection with the microbiome is even less established among the sporty than among the nutrition conscious.

But at least some of these health fans are also interested in the role of their own gut flora. Their point of contact are biotech companies that analyze the interior as a service. A Google search with a combination of keywords like "microbiome" and "sequencing" quickly leads to corresponding addresses and a comparison portal (https://www.mymicrobiome.info/gut-microbiome-test-kits-2020.html). Anyone interested in microbiome analyses and willing to invest about 150 euros in their health can have the species composition of their gut flora determined from a tiny stool sample sent in. The relatively low price is explained by the fact that the customer allows the company to use their anonymized data for research purposes. Via a website, you can retrieve the results and find out the extent to which the frequency of the important bacterial species of your own microbiome is within the normal range or deviates from normal values. At the same time, you receive hints via the website on how to improve your diet and support bacteria that, for example, positively influence digestion, the integrity of the intestinal mucosa, the tendency towards inflammation, calorie utilization, sleep quality or mood.

In some circles, such analyses have become a lifestyle product, because it is good to know more about one's inner life. However, the hints are usually relatively superficial, because the analyses of the 16S rRNA gene, on which they are based, only provide relatively rough information. But at least these analyses end the blind flight in terms of intestinal bacteria that has prevailed so far. With the decline in prices for DNA sequencing and improvements in the algorithms for evaluation, the analyses will certainly become cheaper and more accurate. So, it is probably only a matter of time before microbiome analyses become be part of the regular services paid by statutory health insurances.

Some of the microbiome companies have further developed their business model and offer customers suitable probiotic bacteria and prebiotics based on their personal data. The next step in commercialization would be the establishment of health clubs where you can specifically purchase the suitable pro-, pre-, syn- and psychobiotics, as well as dietary supplements, fitness bracelets, sports equipment and other accessories for a healthy life against the background of your individual genome and microbiome data. Older people, who are more willing and often also financially able to invest in health prevention, could be especially good customers there. It is also conceivable that, in the not-too-distant future, the production of personalized bacterial cocktails will be offered that can beneficially supplement your own microbiome as a gut capsule, skin cream or inhalation spray.

The new ideas from the health scene are inspiring, but only when you have the commensals in view do the individual elements fit together properly and a direction emerges. A lot is gained with a healthy diet. But it is not enough to swallow a few dietary supplements or shop in the organic supermarket, because the sugary lemonades sold there are just as unhealthy as elsewhere. And even if you eat vegan, it may be that fiber and variety are lacking. Sport and exercise are important, but they alone do not guarantee health if the microbiome suffers from a diet of steaks and power drinks.

In addition, the immune system needs challenges to keep its anti-inflammatory mechanisms in shape. Apparently, environmental bacteria are important for this, as they temporarily populate the skin and intestines and trigger alarms with their danger signals, but without causing diseases. The importance of this component is shown by the example of the Irish Travellers: If you spend most of your time outdoors and are constantly surrounded by other people and animals, you apparently remain spared from inflammatory diseases, even if your diet is unhealthy, thanks to a diverse microbiome.

References

Allen JM et al (2017) Exercise training-induced modification of the gut microbiota persists after microbiota colonization and attenuates the response to chemically induced colitis in gnotobiotic mice. Gut Microbes 9:115–130

Ananthakrishnan AN et al (2013) A prospective study of long-term intake of dietary fiber and risk of Crohn's disease and ulcerative colitis. Gastroenterol 145:970–977

Asnicar F et al (2021) Microbiome connections with host metabolism and habitual diet from 1,098 deeply phenotyped individuals. Nat Med 27:321–332

Bay L et al (2020) Universal dermal microbiome in human skin. MBio 11:202945–202919

Bolte LA et al (2021) Long-term dietary patterns are associated with pro-inflammatory and anti-inflammatory features of the gut microbiome. Nat Med 27:31–332

Cook MD et al (2016) Exercise and gut immune function: evidence of alterations in colon immune cell homeostasis and microbiome characteristics with exercise training. Immun Cell Biol 94:158–163

Debarry J et al (2007) Acinetobacter lwoffi and Lactococcus lactis strains isolated from farm cowsheds possess strong allergy protective properties. J Allergy Clin Immunol 119:1514–1521

DGE (2021). https://www.dge.de/ernaehrungspraxis/vollwertige-ernaehrung/10-regeln-der-dge/. Accessed 28 Mar 2021

Fyhrquist N et al (2014) Acinetobacter species in the skin microbiota protect against allergic sensitization and inflammation. J Allergy Clin Immunol 134:1301–1309

Hanski I et al (2012) Environmental biodiversity, human microbiota, and allergy are interrelated. PNAS 109:8334–8339

Harper JW, Zisman TL (2016) Interaction of obesity and inflammatory bowel disease. World J Gastroenterol 21:7868–7881

IARC (2018) Red meat and processed meat. In: IARC monographs on the evaluation of carcinogenic risks to humans, vol 114

Keohane DM et al (2010) Microbiome and health implications for ethnic minorities after enforced lifestyle changes. Nat Med 26:1089–1095

Matsumoto et al (2008) Voluntary running exercise alters microbiota composition and increases n-butyrate concentration in the rat cecum 72:572–78

Mailing LJ (2019) Exercise and the gut microbiome: a review of the evidence, potential mechanisms, and implications for human health. Exerc Sport Sci Rev 47:75–85

Marino E et al (2017) Gut microbial metabolites limit the frequency of autoimmune T cells and protect against type 1 diabetes. Nat Immunol 18:552–562

Menni C et al (2021) High intake of vegetables is linked to lower white blood cell profile and the effect is mediated by the gut microbiome. BMC Med 19:37

Nakatsuji T et al (2013) The microbiome extends to subepidermal compartments of normal skin. Nat Commun 4:1431

National Geographic (2016) https://www.nationalgeographic.com/photography/article/irish-travellers-uphold-the-traditions-of-a-bygone-world. Accessed 3 Mar 2022

Nutrition Council Berlin (2021) Berlin isst anders. www.ernaehrungsrat-berlin.de. Accessed 18 Nov 2021

Roslund MI et al (2020) Biodiversity intervention enhances immune regulation and health-associated commensal microbiota among day-care children. Sci Adv 6:eaba2578

Ruokolainen L et al (2025) Green areas around homes reduce atopic sensitization in children. Eur J Allergy Clin Immunol 70:195–202

Sharif K et al (2018) Physical activity and autoimmune diseases: get moving and manage the disease. Autoimmun Rev 17:53–72

Thorburn AN et al (2015) Evidence that asthma is a developmental origin disease influenced by maternal diet and bacterial metabolites. Nat Commun 6:8320

Vangay P et al (2018) US immigration westernizes the human gut microbiome. Cell 175:962–972

Wagenaar CA et al (2021) The effect of dietary interventions on chronic inflammatory diseases in relation to the microbiome: a systematic review. Nutrients 13:3208

Willet W et al (2019) Food in the anthropocene: the EAT-lancet commission on healthy diets from sustainable food systems. Lancet 393:447–492

Zuo T et al (2020) Alterations in gut microbiota of patients with COVID-19 during time of hospitalization. Gastroenterology 159:944–955

8

Excursus

Contents

Microbiome and Microbiota

What is the "microbiome"? The word refers to the community of microbes, i.e., tiny organisms, that live in and on our bodies. This includes bacteria, viruses, certain fungi, and archaea (primitive single-celled organisms). In this book, I also count parasites among the microbes, although some of them are quite large. The term "microbiome" has become common in everyday language, although its meaning is not entirely clear-cut and the word is used differently depending on the case. The term "biome" in biology refers to the organisms of a habitat, so "microbiome" can refer to the entirety of the microorganisms of a body. This is the sense in which this book uses the word microbiome. We also use the well-established term "flora" (i.e., skin flora, gut flora, etc.) in the same sense, although it is actually a botanical term and the microorganisms discussed here are not plants!

In scientific articles, the microorganisms of a habitat are more often referred to as "microbiota", and the word "microbiome" is used for the entirety of the genes of the organisms living there. Both terms are correct; the important thing is only that one agrees on a consistent use of language. Since one does not necessarily have to distinguish exactly between the organisms and their genes in a popular science text like this one, I have opted for the more common terms "microbiome" and "flora" when referring to the microbial community.

The organisms of the microbiome influence humans in various ways. It is not always clear how close the cohabitation must be for an effect to occur. Even microbes that come from the environment, for example, from dust, soil or untreated water, can influence humans, especially if they survive in the body for a while. Therefore, when talking about the microbiome and its effect on humans, one should not forget the influence of the entire living environment on us.

Bacteria and the Concept of Species

The classification of bacteria into species is fraught with difficulties, because they do not reproduce sexually, but mainly by division. This results in thousands of daughter cells within a short time, so that mutants occur much more frequently than in organisms with slower reproduction. For this reason alone, bacterial populations are genetically diverse. In addition, bacteria have a very flexible genome and exchange DNA with relatives relatively easily. Therefore, the bacteria of a species often differ greatly in terms of their properties. We thus speak of bacterial strains. Well-characterized bacteria such as Escherichia coli (= E. coli) are named according to the classic species designation, which consists of the Latin genus and species names. However, this species encompasses a quite genetically diverse group of bacteria.

In microbiome analyses, the question as to what extent one can or cannot group genetically diverse bacteria into a species is circumvented, and the different bacteria are divided into "operational taxonomic units" (= OTUs). To do this, the DNA sequence of a specific gene, the 16S rRNA gene, of the bacteria in a sample is determined. Bacteria whose sequences of this marker gene match more than 97% are grouped into an OTU. An OTU is, so to speak, a pot into which all closely related bacterial strains are put. Thus, OTUs loosely define close kinship groups of bacteria, much like species do. A new type of grouping into "amplicon sequence variants" (ASVs) is now becoming established, a grouping that works significantly more accurately than OTUs due to built-in error correction.

Not All Farms Are the Same

Children who grew up on a farm have a lower risk of developing allergies and asthma later in life than children from an urban environment. To explore the causes of this difference, one must delve deeper and compare the effect of different farms. Indeed, there is a scientist who has done exactly that. In 2019, I met Prof. Erika von Mutius, a wiry, dynamic pediatrician and director of the Helmholtz Institute for Allergy Prevention in Munich. We chatted in a hotel lobby in downtown Berlin, the interview lasting just under an hour. She had accepted an invitation to speak at the Berlin Museum of Natural History as part of the prestigious lecture series "Science in the Dinosaur Hall", speaking about her work under the tallest dinosaur skeleton in the world. Erika von Mutius is one of the driving forces behind large epidemiological studies on the spread of asthma. In Europe-wide research, she and her colleagues from many countries investigated why children from traditionally operating farms have a lower allergy and asthma risk than children who grew up in the city. In the USA, she found a dream constellation that allowed her to explore the causes of the farm effect.

As she related it to me, Prof, von Mutius, at an international conference in 2010, got into a conversation with an American allergist who told her about his wife, also a doctor and director of a clinic that served people without health insurance in the American state of Indiana, a task she took up out of a sense of social commitment. Given the area, the service was used by many Amish. The Amish are members of a religious community that emerged from the Anabaptist movement whose ancestors, persecuted for their faith, emigrated from German-speaking areas to America. Today, many followers still live there in close religious communities that practice traditional agriculture. Among other things, they reject motorization, so their simple farm machinery is pulled by horses and people travel by carriage. In the clinic, it was noticed that asthma and allergies were virtually non-existent among the Amish—in stark contrast to the typical American population in the same area.

Prof. Mutius, picking up on this thread, decided to visit one of the Amish communities in Indiana. During our interview, she vividly told me how much this visit resembled a journey back in time to her own childhood in the 1950s. in Berchtesgadener Land, when agriculture was still practiced on small farms, many people kept a pig or a goat, or at least rabbits and chickens, and having your own vegetable garden was a given. In the middle of the USA, she says, life among the Amish still goes on today much as it used to in the village where her aunt lived, and where she would visit during the holidays: The mostly large families live on farms consisting of residential buildings, stables, and barns. The cowsheds are located in the immediate vicinity of the apartments, so there is constant contact with the animals. The children participate in the life and work of the adults. The food mostly comes from their own operations. In addition, there is a constant coming and going, with visits by neighbors and numerous relatives being an essentially permanent state. So, this is what an environment looks like where asthma and allergies are virtually unknown!

Erika von Mutius had found the perfect control group for thoroughly investigating the causes of the quasi-absence of allergic diseases among the Amish. Another religious community that immigrated from Europe to the USA, the Hutterites, also practice agriculture, but have adopted many elements of modern life. They originally come from Tyrol, and, like the Amish, also sought refuge in the USA for religious reasons. The original homelands of these two European ethnic groups are only about 150 km apart. In their new homeland, both kept to themselves and did not mix with the rest of the population. Thus, Amish and Hutterites are both still very genetically similar today to what they had been, an important prerequisite for the comparability of results.

Unlike the Amish, the Hutterites practice mechanized agriculture on a large scale, work with modern methods, and have barns for up to 100,000 turkeys, 20,000 pigs, or 600 cattle. They live in colonies of houses that are located at a greater distance from the barns, so, as a Hutterite, you have little contact with the animals except at work. In addition, unlike the Amish, Hutterite culture excludes women and girls from barn work.

These differences in economy and culture are associated with very different rates of allergic diseases: 5.2% of Amish children from Indiana had mostly mild symptoms of asthma and 7.2% showed a predisposition to allergies in blood tests. In contrast, these figures were about four times higher for Hutterite children from South Dakota, at 21.3% and 33.3%, respectively (Ober et al.

2017). Tests also showed that the immune system of Amish children had reached a state of tolerance, so that harmless substances did not trigger significant inflammatory reactions. Apparently, the modern lifestyle of the Hutterite children had led to a significantly increased disease rate.

Further investigations by the working group of Prof. von Mutius showed that the cause of the tolerance of Amish children was the constant inhalation of bacteria-laden dust from their environment. Where barns are in close proximity, flies buzz around and there is a constant coming and going of people, dogs and cats, there are more and different bacteria in the dust than in a normal household. Therefore, the traditional farming lifestyle of the Amish, which corresponds to the rural life of the pre-war period in Europe, protects against allergic diseases! In contrast, meticulous cleanliness, which minimizes contact with bacteria, prepares the ground for an overreaction of the immune system. Most other inflammatory diseases follow the same pattern: Under simple living conditions, as they still prevail in nature-oriented societies or in some regions of developing countries, allergies, asthma, chronic intestinal inflammations, multiple sclerosis, celiac disease and similar ailments are virtually unknown.

Biologics, a Revolution in the Treatment of Inflammatory Diseases

At the end of the 1980s, so-called "biologicals" were developed for the therapy of inflammatory diseases; these are biologically produced molecules, mostly monoclonal antibodies, which have revolutionized treatment. These molecules bind, with high specificity, to their target structure, and thus block it. An important target of these agents is TNF-α, a cytokine with various inflammation-promoting properties.

TNF-α is mainly produced by phagocytes and activates other immune cells to divide and release further cytokines. It not only acts locally, but also on the whole body, switching the metabolism to emergency operation, so that both fat reserves and muscles are broken down. In addition, it contributes to the development of fever, sleep and pain, among other things, and is closely related to the typical symptoms of fatigue. TNF-α is not only important in rheumatoid arthritis, but also plays a crucial role in inflammatory bowel diseases and psoriasis. The development of a new generation of drugs that can switch off such a central messenger substance without massive side effects was not only a pioneering achievement, but also financially very lucrative. Therefore, it is worth taking a closer look at the history of TNF blockers.

The first TNF-α blocker was a monoclonal antibody named Infliximab. It was developed in 1989 by Jan Vilcek and Junming Le, two scientists at the Medical Faculty of New York University. Monoclonal antibodies are produced by immunizing a mouse with a substance, in our case, TNF-α, and then fusing its antibody-producing cells, the B cells, with tumor cells. With a suitable selection process, cells can then be identified that proliferate indefinitely like tumor cells and, at the same time, produce antibodies like B cells and secrete them into the cell culture fluid. Vilcek and Le went a step further and altered part of the antibody molecule using biotechnical methods, making Infliximab more tolerable for patients.

The first patient to be treated was a 16-year-old girl in an Amsterdam hospital; she had inflammatory bowel disease and did not respond to medication. The success was sensational, as the clinical picture had normalized after just 1 week. The product was first approved in the USA in 1998, for the treatment of Crohn's disease, under the brand name "Remicade". Just 1 year later, it was approved in the USA for rheumatoid arthritis, the largest market for the drug, and for other inflammatory diseases. Given the high number of chronically ill people, the demand for the new active ingredient was enormous, despite the high costs that such a product produced in cell culture causes. Remicade became a "blockbuster" among drugs and is still on the market today.

The driving force behind the development of Remicade was the immunologist Jan Vilcek. He was born in 1933—the year Hitler came to power—in what is now Slovakia. As the child of Jewish parents, Vilcek was fortunate to survive fascism. He studied medicine in Czechoslovakia, became interested in immunology and cytokines from an early age, and defected to the USA with his wife in 1965. The Medical Faculty of New York University immediately offered him a scientist position without any formalities. There, he delved into research, receiving numerous patents. The development of Remicade was therefore no accident. However, no one would have guessed that it would be such an economic success. The drug brought in billions, of which the inventors also had a share. Jan Vilcek and his wife Marica, however, stuck to their unpretentious lifestyle, founding the Vilcek Foundation in 2000, an organization that donates significant financial support to science and the arts.

The world's biggest blockbuster in the pharmaceutical industry is now the human anti-TNF-a antibody Adalimumab (trade name "Humira"), which is produced using molecular biological methods and which treats rheumatoid arthritis (RA) and other inflammatory diseases. Humira was developed by the German company BASF and is distributed by the American pharmaceutical company Abbvie. RA patients with severe progression must inject the antibody every 2 weeks, often for years or decades. A dose cost about 445 euros in Germany in 2022, resulting in annual costs of more than 11,000 euros per patient for the drug alone. Compared to the drugs of the previous generation, these are astronomical sums, but they are justified by the high development and manufacturing costs—and not least by the success. In 2021 alone, Humira brought Abbvie a worldwide turnover of 20.69 billion US dollars (Statista 2021)! With such sums, it is understandable that health insurance companies urge a sparing use of biologics, as the high costs threaten to overwhelm the health systems.

After the patents for the first approved biologics expired, such as in the case of Humira in 2018, more and more copycat products, so-called "biosimilars", began appearing on the market. As TNF blockers, all these drugs have a comparably far-reaching effect. However, their side effects are also similar, as they all directly intervene in the immune system. Immunosuppression through the elimination of TNF-a implies an efficiency loss of immune responses, so that certain viral diseases, such as influenza or hepatitis, and chronic infections with some bacteria can run more virulently. In particular, the blockade of TNF-a in the early stages of treatment led to the flare-up of tuberculosis in patients with silent infection, so that, today, it is routine to check patients for whether or not they carry this infection.

Innate and Acquired Immune System

Not only does our human genome carry the heritage of our primate ancestors, it also reflects the more distant past when the globe was only inhabited by invertebrates. That's why we actually have two immune systems that work very well together. Both systems consist of billions of independent individual cells, the white blood cells. Most of these immune cells are quite mobile and migrate with blood and lymph fluid throughout the body. They are concentrated in certain organs, such as the intestine, lymph nodes, bone marrow, spleen, and thymus. They communicate with each other through messenger substances and physical contacts.

From the primordial crabs and insects comes a rather simple, so to speak, analog system, which immediately goes into attack mode when it recognizes certain foreign structures. How one then reacts is genetically determined, which is why we speak of the innate immune system. Vertebrates have also developed a sophisticated, programmable system that recognizes all conceivable molecular structures through adaptation: the adaptive immune system. It takes a longer time to get started when it first comes into contact with foreign substances, but it develops a memory, and can then react very quickly and efficiently when repeated contact occurs. What has only recently become known: The adaptive immune system not only attacks inflammatory responses, but also very efficiently suppresses them.

The most important cells of the innate immune system are various types of phagocytes. They can best be compared to amoebas, tiny single-celled organisms that can change their shape, move in a targeted crawling manner, and flow around food particles. In a very similar way, phagocytes take up bacteria or cell debris that they recognize with their receptors. If they encounter signals indicating pathogens, they are activated, attack the invaders with aggressive chemicals, and attract more immune cells with messenger substances. This results in inflammation within a few hours.

The acquired immune system is mainly based on B and T cells, whose receptors are randomly assembled. They can therefore recognize any possible molecular structure. When the cells recognize a substance with their receptors for the first time, they are activated, divide massively, and produce cytokines that control other immune cells. It takes several days for the reaction to be fully developed. During this time, long-lived memory cells also form, so that the acquired immune system reacts faster through repeated recognition. The B cells carry antibodies as receptors on their surface and release large amounts of these molecules into the body fluids. The T cells carry receptors on their surface that recognize fragments of proteins. These fragments must be presented to them by other cells (usually phagocytes) along with additional signals as if on a silver platter. For this presentation, each person has different sets of molecules, the HLA proteins (HLA for "Human Lymphocyte Antigen").

The additional signals during the presentation program the T cell and its offspring and determine whether they are stimulating or producing inhibitory neurotransmitters. In the context of immune tolerance, regulatory T cells ("Tregs") are of particular interest, as they suppress inflammatory processes with their cytokines and calm the immune system. The most efficient of these inhibitory cytokines is IL-10, which lays a veritable fire blanket over the hotbed of inflammation.

Macro- and Micronutrients

A Little Carbohydrate Science

Carbohydrates do not have the best reputation. They are commonly considered to be fattening. Therefore, low-carb diets are currently booming among figure-conscious health enthusiasts. Even evolution is used as a justification: Because humans only came to grains and potatoes relatively late, our digestive system is much more adapted to meat and fish, say the advocates of the Paleolithic and other diets. This is not necessarily correct, as the few hunter-gatherers still existing today live predominantly on plant food, which consists largely of carbohydrates. And it is very likely that many of our ancestors had a similar diet. Moreover, in societies that lived predominantly on meat, fat and fish, such as the Inuit in polar regions, the rate of diet-related diseases was very high, which argues against a diet without carbohydrates.

All carbohydrates have in common that they are made up of sugar molecules or saccharides and are the most important energy source for most animals and humans. However, there are huge differences between carbohydrates. For our purposes, we can roughly distinguish between (1) carbohydrates that are directly digested by humans, (2) carbohydrates that are broken down in the intestine by bacteria and (3) those that pass through the digestive system undigested. In addition, there is the accessibility of the carbohydrates: Are they enclosed in plant cells that first need to be cracked by bacteria (as in whole grain bread) or are they freely accessible (as in white bread)?

The carbohydrates directly digestible by humans include the simple sugars (monosaccharides) such as glucose (dextrose) and fructose (fruit sugar). Their molecules are small, and are therefore quickly absorbed into the blood in the small intestine. Glucose serves all body cells as their most important fuel and provides immediate energy, while fructose is converted into fat in the liver and stored as an energy reserve.

These single molecules can also be combined in pairs, in which case they are called disaccharides. This includes the most commonly used household sugar or crystal sugar, the sucrose. It consists of one molecule of glucose and one molecule of fructose and is made from sugarcane or beet juice. Therefore, cane sugar is chemically no different than beet sugar. Disaccharides must be broken down into the single molecules by digestive enzymes before they can be absorbed in the small intestine. Mono- and disaccharides are referred to as "sugar" on food packaging, and the term is used in this way here as well.

Sugar is an important energy provider, with the brain being the biggest glucose consumer of them all. Therefore, evolution has trained us to love sugar and eat a lot of sweets. However, it did not consider that Homo sapiens could ever suffer from abundance. An excess of glucose leads to obesity, with all its negative consequences, and to type 2 diabetes and tooth decay. The fact that these evils are so widespread is partly due to the fact that sugar is ubiquitous in foods. Apart from breakfast cereals, chocolate and desserts, which we know contain sugar, it is hidden in many foods to increase their attractiveness. Even pickles, sausage and packet soups contain hidden sugars. As the body quickly gets used to the taste and wants more, consumption can easily increase, which increases sales. However, the taste buds can be readjusted if we use sugar only when something is actually supposed to taste sweet. Those who cook fresh meals themselves have control over the consumption of sugar and can reduce it.

The trend today is moving away from sucrose to isoglucose, usually indicated as fructose-glucose syrup, which is increasingly replacing conventional sugar. This sugar syrup is usually chemically produced from corn starch and is therefore much cheaper than cane sugar. In the USA, this "high fructose corn syrup" already accounts for about 50% of the sugar consumed there. The chemical components of isoglucose (55% fructose, 45% glucose) are present in a ratio similar to that of household sugar, so its use is not a concern from a medical point of view. However, since the molecules are already separated, they are absorbed even more efficiently by the upper small intestine than those of cane sugar and cause a shift of energy into the fat stores. Thus, isoglucose is likely to further intensify the already existing trend towards overweight (Fig. 8.1).

Molecules composed of more than two individual sugars are called oligosaccharides, while large complexes of many individual sugars are called polysaccharides. The most important polysaccharide in regard to nutrition is starch. It is found, for example, in cereal grains and potatoes and is made up of tens of thousands of glucose molecules. Most forms of starch are broken down into individual glucose molecules by human enzymes and then absorbed by the small intestine. If starch is, for example, enclosed in plant cells or biochemically altered so that it cannot be broken down by the intestine, it is referred to as digestion-resistant starch. This passes through the small intestine and can then be broken down in the large intestine by bacteria, which use whole batteries of enzymes for this purpose.

In addition to digestion-resistant starch, many other polysaccharides are indigestible for human enzymes, but good fodder for intestinal bacteria. This includes inulin, a polysaccharide made up of fructose units that is stored by plants such as chicory, artichokes and Jerusalem artichokes as an energy reserve. Other plant polysaccharides are fructans and pectin, which are contained in fruits and vegetables. Even polysaccharides like the wood component cellulose can be cracked by certain bacteria of the intestinal flora. The bacteria in the large intestine break down these substances into individual sugars, which they then utilize themselves, because hardly any sugar is absorbed into the body down there. The benefit for humans is the short-chain fatty acids that are produced during the breakdown, which will be mentioned further below.

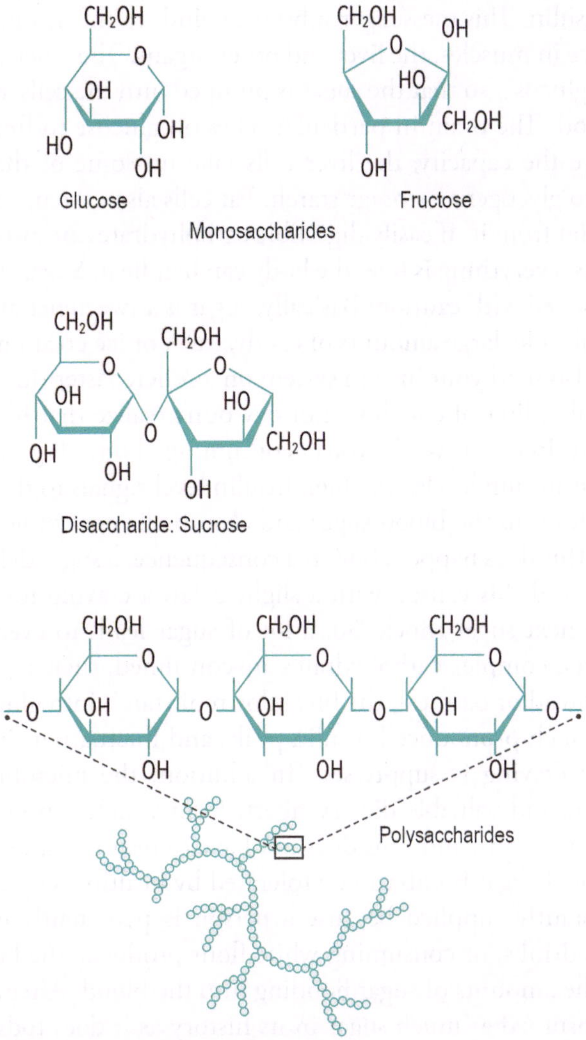

Fig. 8.1 Comparison of sugar molecules—glucose, fructose, sucrose, polysaccharides. (© Scorpio Verlag in Europa Verlage GmbH, München. Reproduced with permission)

Danger from Sugar Bombs

As already mentioned, the health effects of carbohydrates also depend on how they are present in a food. Easily accessible carbohydrates, i.e., sugar (= mono and disaccharides) and digestible starch are broken down into individual sugars in the small intestine and quickly absorbed into the blood. When the glucose level in the blood rises after a sugary meal, the pancreas responds by producing insulin. This messenger substance binds to the insulin receptors on the cell surface in muscles, the liver and other organs. This opens the transport channels for glucose, so that the sugar is pumped into the cells and disappears from the blood. The brain in particular relies on glucose to function well. If they still have the capacity, the liver cells take up some of the glucose and convert it into glycogen, a storage starch. Fat cells also take up sugar and produce storage fat from it. If easily digestible carbohydrates are available in moderate amounts, everything is fine, the body can handle it. Sugar itself, however, should be enjoyed with caution: Basically, sugar is a sweetener and not a food.

Sugar bombs like large amounts of candy, cake, or ice cream not only make you fat, but also send your insulin system on a rollercoaster ride. Most people who drink half a liter of cola on a hot day don't realize that it's a 10 percent sugar solution. In other words, you're consuming about 50 g of sugar, which drives up your insulin levels. The high insulin level signals to the body cells to thoroughly clean up the blood sugar and absorb all sugar molecules into the cell interior. This does happen, but, as a consequence, a sugar deficiency in the blood arises. And this causes, with a slight delay, a craving for more sweets, and thus the next sugar shock. So, a lot of sugar leads to even more sugar. However, when complex carbohydrates are consumed, such as in the form of whole grain bread or oatmeal, the breakdown of starch into glucose is slower. There are no such pronounced insulin peaks and fluctuations in blood sugar levels, so the craving is suppressed. In addition, the microbiome receives micronutrients and valuable dietary fibers, from which it produces calming short-chain fatty acids, and thus does not have to resort to intestinal mucus.

An occasional sugar bomb can be tolerated by healthy people. However, if sugar is constantly supplied because a person is persistently eating sweets, drinking soft drinks, or consuming white flour products, the body cells cannot process the amounts of sugar flooding into the blood. After all, humanity has never consumed as much sugar in its history as it does today. Under the overload, the insulin receptors become dull and the cells become "insulin resistant", meaning they no longer respond, even if the pancreas increases the output of insulin. But since the intestine has no built-in brake and continues to absorb as much sugar as possible, there are constantly elevated blood sugar levels. This gradually leads to type 2 diabetes, the most common form of diabetes. Too much sugar in the blood and body fluids then leads to damage to the blood vessel and nervous systems with a multitude of subsequent diseases. The medical literature is full of images of common consequences, namely, poorly healing wounds and amputated toes. Formerly referred to as "old age diabetes", the disease is now increasingly occurring in adolescents. Risk factors are overweight and lack of exercise, but also genetic predispositions. If the disease is not too advanced, the most effective therapy is a change in diet. Avoiding simple carbohydrates, consuming fewer calories and engaging in a lot of exercise are then the most important advice from the doctor.

Dietary Fiber: Food for the Bacteria

The polysaccharides that humans cannot digest are referred to as dietary fiber. This food component has long been neglected, but is extremely valuable! It was already known that dietary fiber promotes digestion by stimulating bowel activity, binding water, and thus giving the stool its consistency. But dietary fiber is also a source of short-chain fatty acids, which are produced by certain types of bacteria during the breakdown of plant substances. The small molecules, which include acetic acid, propionic acid, and butyric acid, have a strong smell and are slightly volatile. Anyone who has ever smelled rancid butter knows what I'm talking about. However, butyric acid & Co. are used by intestinal cells or in the liver as a source of energy. In this way, they contribute about 10% of human calories. In times of scarcity, this can be a vital asset.

Another function of short-chain fatty acids cannot be overestimated: They are calming pills for the immune system. If suitable bacteria are present, the molecules they release inhibit inflammatory reactions. Butyric acid is particularly efficient in this respect. It acts on dendritic cells, which lie directly beneath the intestinal epithelium (Fig. 4.6 in the book). When they sense butyric acid with their receptors, they influence the development of control cells of the immune response, the T cells. Under the influence of dendritic cells, they develop into regulatory T cells or Tregs. As already mentioned earlier, these cells and their descendants recognize foreign substances, but rather than triggering inflammation, they inhibit it. As the peacekeeping forces of the immune system, they prevent irrelevant irritations or errors in the system from immediately turning into inflammation.

Since 70% of immune cells are located near the intestine, the short-chain fatty acids produced in the intestine influence the entire immune system. The discovery of this connection by the laboratory of nutritionist Wendy Garrett from the Harvard School of Public Health in Boston (Smith et al. 2013) has been enormously influential to nutrition research. To ensure an adequate supply of short-chain fatty acids, a balanced diet rich in dietary fiber is important.

Dietary fiber from whole grain products, legumes, nuts, seeds, fruits, and vegetables ensures that the bacteria species that grow are those that dampen inflammatory reactions with their short-chain fatty acids. Each plant species has its own variety of dietary fiber. One roughly distinguishes between soluble dietary fibers, such as fructans, pectins, and ß-glucans from fruits and vegetables, and insoluble ones such as cellulose and lignin. For each of these substances, there are specialists in the microbiome that split large molecules into smaller ones or utilize the resulting waste products. The more varied the diet, the greater the number of specialized bacterial species involved in the breakdown of dietary fiber and the supply of short-chain fatty acids.

How very specific dietary fibers influence immune responses, and thus inflammatory diseases, via the microbiome is shown by a study involving mice. If cellulose, the most common polysaccharide found in the cell wall of plants, was missing in the animals' feed, the microbiome of the animals changed and they developed chronic intestinal inflammation. The frequency of the intestinal bacterium Alistipes feingoldii decreased most significantly. However, when the mice were then specifically colonized with this bacterium, the tendency towards intestinal inflammation decreased (Fischer et al. 2020). Cellulose is therefore not a neutral molecule in mice—as is very likely also the case in humans—but has an important function in maintaining the immunological balance.

A large variety of dietary fibers, as recommended by nutrition physiologists, ensures that the bacterial flora is also rich in species. This diversity is an important safeguard against crises: If, for example, some bacterial species are decimated by necessary antibiotic treatment or an infection, other, similar species can take over their job and, for example, step in in the production of short-chain fatty acids. However, if dietary fibers are neglected in the diet, the bacteria starve and have to resort to the carbohydrate-rich mucus that lines the colon as emergency rations. This meager food produces fewer short-chain fatty acids, and thus fewer calming pills for the immune system. In addition, a thin, gnawed mucus layer only very imperfectly shields the intestine from pathogens and its own intestinal bacteria, thus promoting inflammation.

Fat and Fat Are Not the Same

Fats (scientifically: "lipids") have gotten very bad press for decades. Avoidance of fats was the health recipe par excellence. Low-fat products and diet margarine were bestsellers. This simple view has always been too short-sighted, because a life without fats is simply impossible. Fats serve as fuel, but they are also, above all, the most important building blocks of cell membranes, making up the semi-liquid shells that surround all of our cells. Moreover, the body can only absorb the vital vitamins A, D, E, and K with the help of fats. There are even several "essential" fatty acids, without which deficiencies occur. They must be taken in with food and are the starting material for important signal molecules that can regulate inflammation and even the feeling of hunger. In this sense, fats are actually health boosters—if the right ones are enjoyed. Sweden was the first Western country to change its national dietary guidelines, in 2013, recommending a diet that is "low carb—high fat", after a health commission published summary results from 16,000 studies (Swedish Council on Health Technology Assessment 2013).

Fats in foods are thus being rehabilitated, but it would be an exaggeration to elevate them to diet heaven in a general sense. There are two reasons for this: First, there are very large differences between fats, which I will discuss further below. Second, it must be considered that fats are the most calorie-rich nutrients and contain more than twice as many calories per gram as carbohydrates or proteins. Where many calories are involved, there is a risk of obesity. And obesity is a risk factor for heart disease, type 2 diabetes and many other ailments, including inflammatory diseases.

Storage fat under the skin, the oft-mentioned "love handles", may disturb our sense of aesthetics, but it is relatively harmless. Really harmful, on the other hand, are fat deposits that are stored in the abdominal cavity: the so-called visceral fat, or fat deposits in the liver and muscles. Fat cells in these regions produce adipokines, i.e., inflammation-promoting hormones. In addition, macrophages also migrate into this adipose tissue, the body's most effective phagocytes, and release inflammation-promoting messenger substances. Therefore, visceral fat promotes chronic inflammation. The effect of the fat pads can even reach the brain, where, in many overweight people, the hypothalamus, an important control center, becomes inflamed (Kreutzer et al. 2017). This change hinders appetite regulation and promotes obesity, and thus further inflammation (Jais and Brüning 2017).

So, anyone who claims that fatty food makes you slim is wrong. But: Calories are not the only determinant of the quality of fats. To understand this, one must deal a little more with the chemical structure. Don't worry, it's not complicated. The vast majority of fats taken in with food consist of triglycerides (somewhat outdated "neutral fats"), which are composed of a molecule of glycerin and three (= tri) fatty acid molecules. One can imagine a triglyceride as a fork with three prongs (Fig. 8.2). Triglycerides from food are split in the small intestine, transported as individual components through the intestinal wall, reassembled in the blood and finally packaged to then reach the place of consumption.

Fats can also exist in the form of unbound fatty acids. These are chains of usually 2–24 carbon atoms, which are linked by single or double bonds.

Further bonding sites are occupied with hydrogen atoms and the ends of the chains carry oxygen atoms. The length of the carbon chains and the number of double bonds determine whether fatty acids are liquid or solid. As a rule of thumb: the longer the chain, the more solid, and the more double bonds there are, the more liquid. The smallest, and therefore most liquid, fatty acids are the beneficial short-chain fatty acids, which are produced by bacteria and apply the brake on inflammation.

A distinction is made among saturated, monounsaturated, polyunsaturated and trans fatty acids. "Saturated" means that all carbon atoms of a fatty acid chain are occupied with hydrogen atoms. In this case, the molecule is evenly built and the chain is straight like a matchstick. Animal-based foods like butter and meats, whether fresh or processed like bacon, are rich in triglycerides with saturated fatty acids. Consumed in excess, these are rather questionable for health, as they are quite efficiently converted into storage fat. This fat then is important, as mentioned above, due to the production of inflammation-promoting messengers (Fig. 8.2).

The long-chain saturated fatty acids are particularly adept at promoting inflammation. In rodents who had had large amounts of them mixed into their food, inflammation values increased just 3 days after the start of the

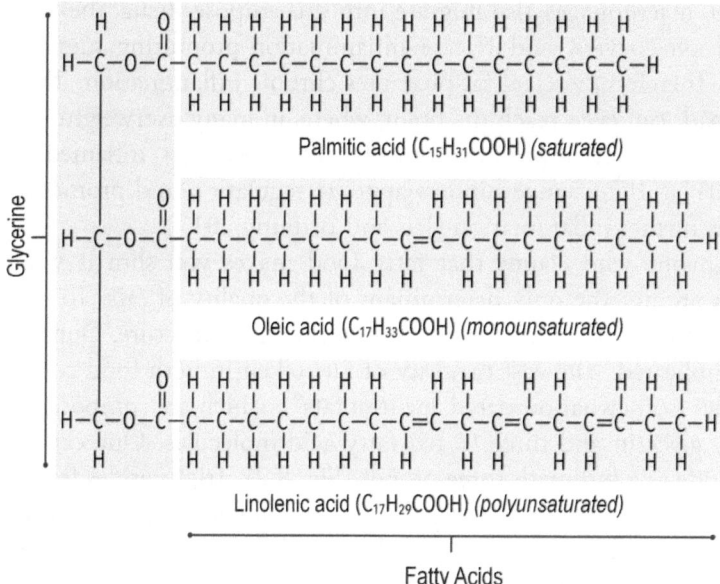

Fig. 8.2 Triglyceride with various fatty acids. (© Scorpio Verlag in Europa Verlage GmbH, München. Reproduced with permission)

experiment. On the other hand, if mice with a disease similar to multiple sclerosis were fed with short-chain fatty acids, their condition improved.

Unsaturated fatty acids are important for a healthy diet. With these fatty acids, which are mainly produced by plants, some carbon atoms of the chain are linked together by double bonds, and therefore cannot bind hydrogen. At these points, the chain creates a bend. Similar to a bent matchstick, not only does the shape change, but the molecule becomes more flexible. If there is only one double bond in the molecule, we speak of monounsaturated fatty acids.

Good sources of monounsaturated fatty acids are, for example, olive oil, nuts, avocados, and poultry meat, but also fatty cold-water fish. Polyunsaturated fatty acids have several of these bends, and therefore have an irregular structure. The position of the bends, denoted by omega, determines the properties. Omega-3 and Omega-6 fatty acids are the most well-known of these because of their health benefits. They are found in sea fish such as mackerel, herring, and salmon, but also in some plants, like rapeseed. The ratio of saturated to unsaturated fats is crucial for a healthy diet. An optimal ratio is 1:2.

The different structure of the fatty acids plays a major role in the construction of cell membranes. These thin shells, which surround each of our cells like an elastic, semi-liquid film, consist of about 90% lipids. Membrane areas with many unsaturated fatty acids are less densely packed due to the irregular structure of the molecules, and are therefore relatively fluid. In contrast, membrane regions with tightly packed saturated fatty acids—much like a bundle of matchsticks—are relatively rigid.

The rigid areas float like islands in the almost liquid areas of the membrane. Sensors and transport proteins are anchored on these islands, which pump sugar, protein building blocks, or other molecules into the cells. A diet rich in unsaturated fatty acids ensures that the cell surface is flexible and that the islands can move well, so that the cell is well supplied.

This flexibility of the cell surface is particularly important in the eyes and the brain, where communication between cells is very intense. Quite surprisingly, the composition of the membrane fatty acids affects very basic processes. For example, in a study at the Berlin Charité, test subjects aged between 50 and 75 years were given fish oil capsules with Omega-3 fatty acids, which make cell membranes flexible, for half a year. At the end of the experiment, the test subjects performed significantly better at thought tasks than the control group. Even more astonishing was the discovery that the brains of the people in the fish oil group had not shrunk, while the control group showed the usual age-related brain volume loss of 0.5%. In some brain regions, the brain structure had even rejuvenated, so there are good reasons to provide yourself with sufficient Omega-3 fatty acids (Witte et al. 2014).

But some omega-3 and omega-6 fatty acids are not only important as a building block for cell membranes, but also as a basic substance for hormones, which is why we—need to ingest them with food, similar to vitamins. Omega-3 fatty acids are especially adept at causing the body to produce lipid hormones that have an anti-inflammatory effect by blocking an important switching mechanism in phagocytes, and thus shutting down their inflammatory program. The starting material for such anti-inflammatory omega-3 fatty acids is alpha-linolenic acid (ALA), which is contained in certain plant oils, especially flaxseed oil. Olive oil, walnuts and chia seeds also contain this important substance.

ALA is converted in the body into the active, anti-inflammatory fatty acid molecules. However, we can also directly absorb the highly effective end products: the actual producers of these health boosters are algae. Through the food chain, the lipids accumulate in larger quantities in cold-water fish such as herring, mackerel and salmon. The fish need omega-3 fatty acids as softeners, so to speak, to keep their cell membranes flexible at cold temperatures. These acids then come onto the market as fish oil. However, one can also buy the anti-inflammatory products in a vegan version, without the detour via the fish, as supplements made from algae are also now on the market.

Messenger substances from omega-6 fatty acids are, rather, pro-inflammatory. They are abundant in most plant oils, such as corn germ, sunflower and soybean oil, and also in animal fats. These fatty acids, unfavorable from an inflammation perspective, include arachidonic acid, which is found in pork fat, for example. However, we need both omega-3 and omega-6 fatty acids, which must be present in a balanced ratio. In the conventional European diet, the ratio of omega-3 to omega-6 fatty acids is about 1:10, but the optimal ratio, according to the WHO, is about 1:5.

Trans fats are only present in small amounts in natural foods, including milk. They are considered unhealthy and pro-inflammatory and increase the risk of heart attacks and strokes. For the food industry, they are made from cheap plant oils through a chemical hardening process. In this process, the bent matchstick of an unsaturated fatty acid is also twisted. The hardening makes fats stiffer, which is how margarine is made from vegetable oil.

Trans fats are found in margarine, chips, puff pastry and other baked goods and sweets. They are used because they are cheap and have a creamy to stiff consistency, without which a cream cake is hardly conceivable. Trans fats are also produced during the processing of fats, for example, by strong heat. So, if the fat in the deep fryer is not changed frequently, the fries not only taste bad, but the health risk also increases. Although manufacturers have now responded to the criticism of their products and have significantly reduced the proportions of trans fats in margarine, for example, one should avoid foods that contain hardened fats.

Proteins

Proteins are among the most important basic building blocks of every cell and make up about 50% of the dry weight of animal cells. In plant cells, the weight proportion is lower because of the often thick cell wall. This also means that, when you think of proteins, you should think beyond such items as steak, because plants also contain proteins, even if they are composed somewhat differently there.

Unlike carbohydrates or fats, proteins cannot be stored by the body in larger quantities. For the construction, maintenance and renewal of body cells, one is therefore dependent on a constant supply of protein. Since cells are constantly renewing, it is difficult to do without proteins for a longer period of time. Because of this constant need, proteins are the most important limiting factor for growth and reproduction. Consumption is particularly high during the growth phase, i.e., in small children, and in pregnant and breastfeeding women. Adults need about 1 g of protein per kg of body weight daily. The diet in industrialized countries usually contains far more than this minimum, therefore protein deficiency is extremely rare here.

A particularly important consumer of proteins is the immune system: Every day, it produces billions of cells and lets the majority of them perish again, only to recycle them. During inflammatory processes, there is an increased need for protein to support the division of immune cells and to produce antibodies, cytokines, and signaling proteins. If there is no supply from outside, the body breaks down muscle mass to meet the protein requirement. In nature, proteins are scarce and in high demand, therefore they are fiercely contested and are essentially the hard currency of life. Whoever can incorporate a lot of protein can grow and reproduce, thus following the ultimate call of evolution.

Proteins consist of long chains of amino acids; often, thousands of these building blocks are linked together like beads (Fig. C). During digestion, the bonds between the beads are broken and the amino acids are absorbed by the intestine and combined into new proteins in the cells. The chains are wound into highly complex tangles, form certain structures or are organized as fibers.

I am most impressed by the proteins that act as enzymes—small molecular machines—that perform the most absurd tasks in the cell, such as the duplication of DNA strands. These must be absolutely precisely constructed in order to function. The blueprint for this is in the DNA, and a total of 20 different standard amino acids are used as building materials. As in a building block system, each of these amino acids has a very specific shape and specific properties. Therefore, to build a certain protein, there must be a sufficient amount of the required amino acids available. To meet this need, the organism requires a well-stocked pool of amino acids. If only one is missing in the mix, the construction of the corresponding protein stalls and the unused amino acids are converted into fat or sugar and burned. About 10% of the daily calories consumed come from proteins (Fig. 8.3).

Dispensable and Indispensable Amino Acids

There is a problem in stocking the amino acid pool, because humans can indeed build 12 amino acids themselves from basic materials, but must take in 8 "indispensable" (formerly: "essential") ones with food. Methionine,

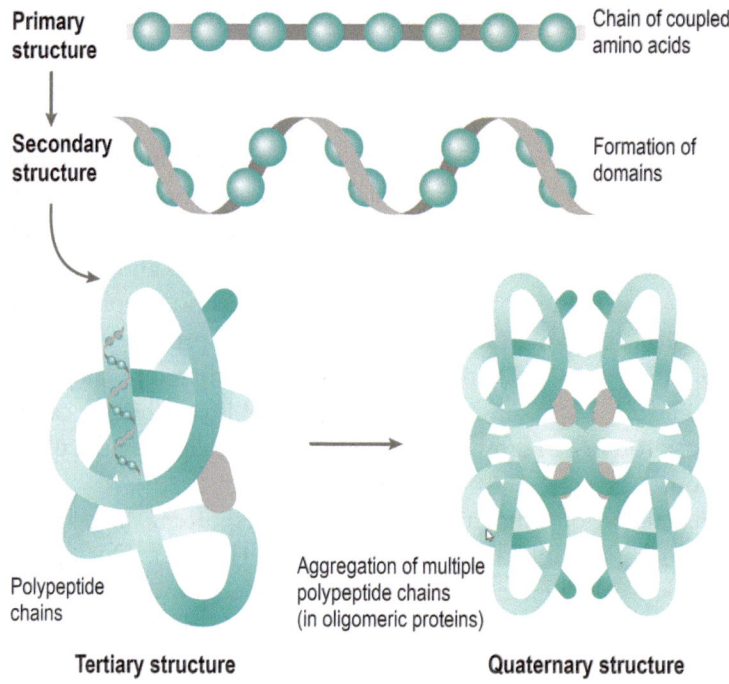

Fig. 8.3 Chains of amino acids form a protein. (© Scorpio Verlag in Europa Verlage GmbH, München. Reproduced with permission)

which serves as the initial building block of every protein, is one of them. Therefore, a lack of methionine can cause the entire protein synthesis, and thus cell division and growth, to stall. Similarly, the other indispensable amino acids limit protein synthesis. Therefore, we must consume enough proteins with our food that the indispensable amino acids like methionine, threonine, and tryptophan never become too scarce.

The proteins of animals contain a spectrum of amino acids similar to those that humans need. Meat, fish, eggs and dairy products usually contain all indispensable amino acids, so our need can be relatively easily met by animal proteins. Plant-based foods can also do this, because legumes, whole grains and nuts are very good suppliers of proteins. However, it should be noted that the proteins of plants usually have an amino acid profile that significantly differs from animal proteins. Therefore, a single plant will usually not provide the full spectrum of indispensable amino acids.

For example, grains contain a lot of methionine, but little tryptophan, lysine, and threonine. Conversely, legumes contain little methionine, but a lot of threonine and tryptophan. Therefore, it is important for vegans to ensure an adequate supply of essential amino acids through the right combination of plant foods. A combination of legumes and cereals would stock the amino acid pool quite well.

In the past, animal proteins were assigned a higher value due to their favorable spectrum of essential amino acids. However, long-term studies have shown that excessive consumption of animal protein can shorten life expectancy, while this is not known to happen with plant protein. In this context, a warning from the World Health Organization made headlines in 2015, declaring, based on large meta-studies, that processed meat is as likely to be carcinogenic as smoking or alcohol consumption (IARC 2018). In addition, red meat, such as beef, pork and lamb, is suspected to be carcinogenic, while fish and poultry were not investigated.

The suspect in the carcinogenicity is not the protein itself, but rather unhealthy additives that are found in foods with animal proteins, for example, if they contain a high proportion of inflammation-promoting saturated fatty acids or have been preserved by pickling or other methods. Carcinogenic pollutants are also produced when grilling, frying and cooking. In the case of red meat, carnitine, a substance that can be broken down into a toxic product in the intestine by the microbiome (see also Chap. 4 on the microbiome in the book), also has a damaging effect. In contrast, plant proteins have additional health benefits, because they come with plant fibers and secondary plant substances.

Because of this important role of proteins, the body must ensure that the supply of amino acids is maintained. To this end, we develop a very specific hunger for protein when the level of essential amino acids drops worryingly. The brain then signals that it is now time to bring in new building material, namely, amino acids. The usual satiety mechanisms are skipped and whatever food is available is eaten in order to grab as much protein as possible. This results in more calories being consumed than are actually necessary for satiety. The result is fat deposits, which support inflammatory diseases, among other things, due to the inflammation-promoting messengers of adipose tissue.

Anyone who wants to live healthily should pay attention to the right mix of protein-rich foods. A well-stocked pool of essential amino acids prevents you from having to eat more than necessary. After consuming junk food and highly processed foods, which usually contain an oversized proportion of carbohydrates and fat, but little protein, the brain quickly signals "hunger" again. Thus, another bag of chips or a piece of cake is consumed, with the known consequences for the scale. With a balanced protein mix, on the other hand, the satiety mechanisms work and it is easier to maintain weight.

Important Vitamins and Minerals

For many metabolic processes, there are vital substances that the body must take in from food. These include vitamins, certain minerals and some secondary plant substances. Nutritionists repeatedly emphasize that a healthy, varied diet covers our need for most of these substances completely.

An exception, however, is vitamin D, a fat-soluble substance that can only be absorbed by the intestine together with fat. The best source is fatty fish (such as herring, mackerel or salmon) or mushrooms and egg yolks. However, most standard diets do not provide sufficient amounts. Fortunately, the body can build up the substance in the skin from inactive precursors itself under the influence of sunlight. However, even in sun-drenched latitudes, only very few people produce sufficient amounts of vitamin D themselves. Therefore, for adequate vitamin D supply, targeted dietary supplementation with appropriate preparations can be useful—especially during the sun-poor winter half-year. To protect children from deficiency, milk is fortified with vitamin D in some countries.

The best-known effect of vitamin D is the regulation of calcium levels in the blood, so it plays an important role in bone formation. However, vitamin D regulates over 1000 genes, including a large number of immune response genes. Among other things, it inhibits one of the most important proteins that transmit inflammation signals within the cell (NFkB), but it also regulates the production of anti-microbial peptides, maintains the intestinal barrier, and influences the composition of the microbiome. Therefore, a deficiency in vitamin D increases the tendency towards inflammation (Zhang et al. 2012a, b). According to a statement by the German Society for Nutrition, 60% of the population falls below the recommended target value of 50 nmol/L in serum (DGE 2012). This value is considered necessary for healthy bone formation. However, the immune-regulating function of vitamin D requires even higher vitamin D levels (Weiss and Litonjua 2017), so, in terms of immune health, an even greater number of Germans would be undersupplied than would be assumed according to the DGE guidelines.

In connection with vitamin D, it is interesting that almost all inflammatory diseases show a north-south gradient of distribution; a typical example would be the increased frequency in Scandinavia compared to Mediterranean countries. According to a common opinion, this increased tendency towards inflammation is associated with the low intensity of sunlight in the north and the consequent lack of vitamin D.

In fact, studies with patients and in animal models show that the UVB component of sunlight raises the vitamin D level and inhibits inflammatory processes. Sunlight therefore has a beneficial effect on inflammatory processes, as long as the dose is not too high. Nevertheless, many epidemiological studies argue against a simple cause-effect relationship (Autier et al. 2017). The equation "a lot of sunlight equals a lot of vitamin D" does not hold up, not least because, in some tropical regions, such as Africa, more people suffer from a deficiency of vitamin D than in the less sunny Western Europe (Mogire et al. 2020).

Moreover, for example, asthma—like other inflammatory diseases—can appear with varied frequency in countries with very similar sun intensity. For example, in Sweden, 20.2% of the population suffers from asthma, while the number in neighboring Finland is significantly lower, at 10.2%. In addition to geographical latitude, factors such as different diets, skin pigmentation, and the duration of time spent outdoors certainly influence vitamin D levels, and thus also the inflammatory process. Since modern humans spend more than 90% of their time indoors, there is still a lot of room for improvement in terms of sunlight.

Vitamin A, which mainly comes from vegetables, liver, and eggs, and is converted in the body into retinoic acid, enhances cell division, and thus supports skin, mucous membranes, bones, cartilage and blood. At the same time, retinoic acid stimulates the formation of regulatory T cells, and thus enhances immune tolerance, but also inhibits infections (Erkelens and Mebius 2017).

Several other vitamins, such as biotin, folic acid, and vitamins B2, B12, and K, are produced by the intestinal flora. In this case, bacterially-produced folic acid is important for humans, while it is unclear whether and to what extent the other vitamins are actually absorbed by the host. Therefore, the role of the microbiome as a vitamin supplier is probably often overestimated.

For balanced immune responses, compounds of the metals zinc and selenium are the most important minerals. Zinc is a component of over 3000 proteins and enzymes, and is therefore a key substance. Compounds of this metal, which are easily absorbed, are found in meat, eggs, milk and seafood. Legumes, nuts, and grain products also contain zinc. However, it is mostly in a bound form, and is more easily absorbed by the body when the products have been sprouted, fermented, or soaked.

Among other things, zinc slows down the activation of immune cells, inhibits enzymes that produce aggressive free radicals, and thus reduces inflammatory responses. Studies in mice suggest that zinc alleviates the symptoms of autoimmune diseases, while, on the other hand, it can enhance allergic reactions (Nishida and Ushida 2018). Selenium, which is mainly found in meat, fish, eggs, and nuts, has a less broad effect, but also inhibits inflammatory responses and protects against free radicals.

Iron is a vital element, with central functions in so many biochemical processes that virtually all organisms need it. It is mainly absorbed from meat, vegetables, and grains. In humans, it is involved in energy production, synthesis of proteins and fats, detoxification, and oxygen transport, but it also has important functions in the production of aggressive molecules, with which the immune response attacks pathogens (and thereby causes collateral damage to its own tissue). But microbes also need iron for their growth!

Given this importance, an efficient defense strategy consists in the scarcity of iron, that is, the body uses all its tricks to bind iron and starve the microbes in relation to the element. The availability of iron is therefore heavily regulated; an excess of it can be harmful and promote infections (Haschka et al. 2021).

Secondary Plant Substances

In addition to vitamins and minerals, secondary plant substances are receiving increasing attention. These substances are not directly vital for plants, but they do, for example, protect them from insect damage or UV radiation, attract pollinators with their scent, or give fruits color. Each plant-based food contains a variety of these substances. For humans, they are particularly important as a component of spices and medicinal herbs, but they also include poisons such as nicotine or the atropine of the deadly nightshade.

Many secondary plant substances are considered healthy, although their effect has only been well documented in a few cases and usually depends on the amount. Too large quantities are toxic in many cases. They work, for example, by binding free radicals, and thus mitigating inflammatory processes, interfering with cellular signaling pathways or inhibiting the growth of certain bacteria. And, of course, they also influence the composition of the gut flora. There are several thousand different secondary plant substances that enter the intestine with food and are broken down and transformed there by the gut bacteria. This results in an immense variety of metabolites that enter the bloodstream and can influence metabolism and the immune and nervous systems.

Well-known secondary plant substances include lycopene, which gives tomatoes and other fruits their red color and acts as a radical scavenger. Another is quercetin, a yellow plant dye that is found in the dye oak, but also in apples, many other fruits, herbs, and vegetables, and that has a similar effect. Blueberries owe their blue color to anti-inflammatory anthocyanins. The glycosinolates, spicy-tasting components of cruciferous vegetables like cabbage and mustard, stimulate DNA repair mechanisms, and thus prevent the development of tumors.

One of the most studied substances is curcumin, the yellow dye from the turmeric root, which also gives Indian curry powder its color and typical flavor. Curcumin also has many other effects, which are controversial.

Secondary plant substances work best in the context of foods, not as isolated substances in pill form, because the best effects are achieved by combinations of several of them at once. The German Society for Nutrition therefore also recommends making use of the variety of vegetables and fruits available and to eat a varied and colourful diet.

Fecal Transplantation

When the inner ecosystem has become so unbalanced that probiotics cannot restore it, gastroenterologists have the transplantation of stool as a last resort. The treatment of severe diarrheal diseases with stool has made a big splash in recent years, especially in alternative circles, but it is not a modern invention, having already been used in China in the fourth century BC (Zhang et al. 2012a, b).

In modern medicine, it has also been rediscovered from time to time. Thus, the journal *The Atlantic* reports that, in 1957, the legendary American microbiologist Stanley Falkow treated patients with their own stool. Severe operations were then prepared with an antibiotic treatment to prevent an infection with hospital pathogens. At the suggestion of his superior, the young assistant, directly after the admission of the sick, had a stool sample taken that was then processed and frozen. After the operation, patients with severe diarrhea were treated by having them swallow gelatin capsules filled with their own stool that released their content in the intestine. When the administrative head of the clinic heard about this, he summoned his innovative colleague and asked him: "Falkow, is it true that you have fed your patients shit?" When the young assistant confirmed this, he was dismissed, but then rehired 3 days later (Blog "Small Things Considered" 2020).

Stool transplants have proven excellent in a situation that often led to death. After antibiotic treatment, in some people can spread the bacterium Clostridium difficile, an otherwise mostly harmless inhabitant of the intestine. As a result, severe, persistent, bloody diarrheal diseases can occur, leading to the death of the patient.

If these clostridia are resistant to antibiotics, and the diarrhea therefore cannot be cured, the person's life is immediately endangered. In patients with this clinical picture, the intestinal ecosystem has been restored by transferring stool from healthy donors. The transplanted bacteria displaced the pathogen and established a new intestinal flora. The cure rate with this method is 90%, a value that is otherwise difficult to achieve with biological methods (Van Nood et al. 2013).

How is stool "transplanted"? The first reaction is to shudder at the thought of handling feces at all. From a medical point of view, however, there is nothing to object to, as long as the transplant does not transmit pathogens. The most important requirement is therefore donors who do not have infections that can be transmitted through feces. Suitable feces are mixed with water and filtered. This liquid is applied by the doctor through a thin tube that goes from the nose through the throat and stomach, directly into the small intestine. Another possibility is to infuse the liquid via the rectal route.

Another method is to administer freeze-dried material in capsules that only dissolve in the small intestine. From there, the bacteria can spread further. It must be ensured that there are enough viable bacteria with the desired positive effect in the transplant. These must be able to assert themselves against the resident microbes and establish themselves in the intestine of the recipient in the long term. After the successes in the treatment of Clostridium difficile infection, the procedure was also tested for other diseases, without a clear picture emerging so far.

A multitude of factors influence the success of stool transplants. For example, recruiting donors from the circle of relatives or from people from the same household can be useful for replenishing a damaged intestinal flora with similar bacteria after an antibiotic treatment. In other cases, ones in which a change in the intestinal flora is desired, stool from people from a foreign environment should be used.

However, it cannot be ruled out that a stool transplant may transmit a disadvantageous intestinal flora to the recipient. Recently, in the USA, following many thousands of positive Clostridium therapies, after an immunosuppressed patient died from an infection with antibiotic-resistant bacteria that was transmitted by a fecal donation, this healing method has come to be viewed very critically (The Atlantic 2019).

References

Autier P et al (2017) Effect of vitamin D supplementation on non-skeletal disorders: a systematic review of meta-analyses and randomised trials. Lancet Diabetes Endocrinol 5:986–1004

Blog "Small Things Considered" (2020). https://schaechterasmblog.org/schaechter/2013/05/fecal-transplants-in-the-good-old-days.html. Accessed 25 Apr 2022

DGE (2012) Deutsche Gesellschaft für Ernährung. https://www.dge.de/wissenschaft/referenzwerte/vitamin-d. Accessed 03 Mar 2022

Erkelens MN, Mebius RE (2017) Retinoic acid and immune homeostasis: A balancing act. Trends Immunol 38:168–180

Fischer F et al (2020) Dietary cellulose induces anti-inflammatory immunity and transcriptional programs via maturation of the intestinal microbiota. Gut Microbes 12:1–17

Haschka D et al (2021) Iron in immune cell function and host defense. Seminars Cell Dev Biol 115:27–36

IARC (2018) Red meat and processed Meat. In: IARC monographs on the evaluation of carcinogenic risks to humans, vol 114

Jais A, Brüning JS (2017) Hypothalamic inflammation in obesity and metabolic disease. J Clin Invest 127:24–32

Kreutzer C et al (2017) Hypothalamic inflammation in human obesity is mediated by environmental and genetic factors. Diabetes 66:2407–2415

Mogire R et al (2020) Prevalence of vitamin D deficiency in Africa: a systematic review and meta-analysis. Lancet Global Health 8:e134–e142

Nishida K, Uchida RU (2018) Role of zinc signaling in the regulation of mast cell-, basophil-, and T cell-mediated allergic responses. J Immunol Res 2018:5749120–5749129

Ober C et al (2017) Immune Development and Environment: Lessons from Amish and Hutterite children. Curr Opin Immunol 48:51–60

Smith PM et al (2013) The microbial metabolites, short-chain fatty acids, regulate colonic Treg homeostasis. Science 341:569–573

Statista (2021). https://de.statista.com/statistik/daten/studie/547194/umfrage/umsatz-des-pharmaunternehmens-abbvie-mit-dem-arzneimittel-humira. Accessed 27 Feb 2022

Swedish Council on Health Technology Assessment (2013) Dietary treatment for obesity. A systematic review of the literature. https://www.dietdoctor.com/swedish-expert-committee-low-carb-diet-effective-weight-loss. Accessed 03 Mar 2022

The Atlantic (2019) Quoted from the blog Small Things considered. https://schaechter.asmblog.org/schaechter/2013/05/fecal-transplants-in-the-good-old-days.html. Accessed 04 Feb 2022

Van Nood E et al (2013) Duodenal infusion of donor feces for recurrent Clostridium difficile. N Engl J Med 368:407–415

Weiss ST, Litonjua AA (2017) Vitamin D in host defense: implications for future research. Am J Respir Cell Mol Biol 56:692–693

Witte AV et al (2014) Long-chain omega-3 fatty acids improve brain function and structure in older adults. Cereb Cortex 24:3059–3068

Zhang Y et al (2012a) Vitamin D inhibits monocyte/macrophage pro-inflammatory cytokine production by targeting MAPK phosphatase-1. J Immunol 188:2127–2135

Zhang F et al (2012b) Should we standardize the 1.700-year-old fecal microbiota transplantation? Am J Gastroenterol 107:1755–1756

Outlook

I hope to have shown in this book that health, in a comprehensive sense, requires the whole package: healthy nutrition, exercise, and contact with nature. Only in this way do we give our inhabitants optimal opportunities to protect us from diseases! It is particularly important that the microbiome be permitted to develop naturally in toddlers, so that the immune system is optimally programmed and the risk of inflammatory diseases later in life decreases. It's fantastic that technical possibilities such as microbiome analysis can be used to inform oneself so as to make the right decisions. In individual cases, probiotics (see Chap. 4) or perhaps even a stool transplantation (see the section "Fecal Transplantation" in Chap. 8) may be offered for microbiome optimization to avoid inflammatory and other diseases. But before one gets into a new loop of consumption, in most cases, it is probably more sensible to first take a moment to pause and consider how one can change one's life in the long term, with healthy nutrition, exercise, and a lot of contact with nature.

R. Lucius, *The Microbiome*, https://doi.org/10.1007/978-3-031-78821-5

Glossary

16S ribosomal RNA RNA, which is a building block of the 16S particles of the bacterial ribosomes. The DNA sequence of the gene is used to differentiate between bacterial species

Actinobacteria A group of gram-positive bacteria; occur mainly in soil

Antigen presentation Presentation of peptides by special proteins on the surface of cells. Enables T cells to recognize these peptides

B cell Cell of the adaptive immune system that produces antibodies

Bacterial transfer Transfer of bacteria into the intestines of mice reared in sterile conditions or treated with antibiotics

Bacteroidetes Phylum of gram-negative bacteria

Bacteroides Class of gram-negative bacteria belonging to the phylum Bacteroidetes; associated to higher consumption of animal-derived proteins

Bifidobacteria An order of bacteria belonging to the phylum Actinobacteria

Blue zone Geographical region in which people reach a remarkably high age; originally marked on a map with a blue ballpoint pen

Celiac disease Inflammatory disease triggered by immune responses against gluten and other components of certain cereals

Commensals Non-harmful inhabitants of a host

Cytokine Messenger molecule of the immune system

Dendritic cell Immune cell with a tree-like structure that efficiently presents peptides on its surface to T cells ("antigen presentation")

Dysbiosis Disruption of the microbiome's balance

Epigenetic modification Changing the accessibility of genes through biochemical processes

Epithel Tissue that covers the surfaces of the body

Escherichia coli Best-known intestinal bacterium; belongs to the phylum Proteobacteria

Fatigue Severe symptoms of exhaustion, caused, among other things, by inflammation-promoting cytokines

Fecal transplantation Transfer of human stool material to another person's gastrointestinal tract to regenerate the microbiome

Fermentation Breakdown of carbohydrates by microorganisms, under exclusion of oxygen

Fiber Dietary substances that cannot be digested by the small intestine; mostly complex carbohydrates

Firmicutes Phylum of predominantly gram-positive bacteria; associated to Western diet

Gram-positive/gram-negative Bacterial cell wall stainable/not stainable by Gram dye. Gram-negative bacteria have a very complex surface structure.

IBD Chronic inflammatory bowel disease

Immune tolerance Ability of the immune system to not react to stimuli via inflammation

Immunological cross-reaction Immune reaction that is triggered by one molecule and also acts on another molecule. For example, antibodies against component A also react against component B if both have a similar molecular structure

Inflammation Activation of immune cells; originally for defense against pathogens

Intestinal barrier The entirety of the intestinal wall, intestinal epithelium and mucus layer. Allows transport of substances, does not allow bacteria to pass through

Leaky gut Permeable intestinal barrier

Macrophage Immune cell, which can have a promoting or inhibiting function in inflammatory processes

Metabolite Product from a metabolic pathway

Microbe Collective term for microorganisms; used here for bacteria, viruses, fungi, archaea, as well as parasitic worms and protozoa

Microbiome Entirety of the microbes colonizing a host organism

Microbiota Term for the microbes of a host organism

MS Multiple sclerosis

Mucus Slimy secrete on the surface of the intestinal epithelium

Phylum In this case a large group of bacteria

Prebiotic Dietary fiber that can be broken down by bacteria

Probiotic Bacteria with health-promoting effect

Proteobacteria Phylum of gram-negative bacteria, often with pro-inflammatory properties

Short-chain fatty acids Fatty acids composed of a small number of carbon atoms, such as acetic acid, butyric acid or propionic acid

Superorganism Entirety of the host and its microbiome

RA Rheumatoid arthritis

T1D Type-1-diabetes

T cell Control cell of the immune system that influences other immune cells via cytokines. There are different forms of T cells: Th1—strongly pro-inflammatory, Th2—less pro-inflammatory, Th17—promote aggressive immune responses, Treg—promote anti-inflammatory immune responses

Treg Regulatory T cell, inhibits inflammation via production of the cytokine IL-10 and other mechanisms

Type 1 diabetes Diabetes caused by destruction of the pancreatic islet cells through autoimmune responses

Visceral fatty tissue Fatty tissue within the abdominal cavity

Western diet Unhealthy diet involving highly processed foods that contain large amounts of simple carbohydrates and fat, but are low in fiber

Western lifestyle Typical lifestyle in industrialized nations, characterized by an unhealthy diet, little exercise and rare contact with nature